MIXED METHODS
RESEARCH

SAGE Mixed Methods Research Series

Vicki L. Plano Clark and Nataliya V. Ivankova,
Series Editors

1. *Mixed Methods in Health Sciences Research: A Practical Primer* by Leslie Curry and Marcella Nunez-Smith

2. *Mixed Methods Research and Culture-Specific Interventions: Program Design and Evaluation* by Bonnie K. Nastasi and John H. Hitchcock

3. *Mixed Methods Research: A Guide to the Field* by Vicki L. Plano Clark and Nataliya V. Ivankova

MIXED METHODS RESEARCH

A Guide to the Field

Vicki L. Plano Clark
University of Cincinnati

Nataliya V. Ivankova
University of Alabama at Birmingham

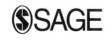

Los Angeles | London | New Delhi
Singapore | Washington DC

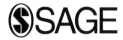

Los Angeles | London | New Delhi
Singapore | Washington DC

FOR INFORMATION:

SAGE Publications, Inc.
2455 Teller Road
Thousand Oaks, California 91320
E-mail: order@sagepub.com

SAGE Publications Ltd.
1 Oliver's Yard
55 City Road
London, EC1Y 1SP
United Kingdom

SAGE Publications India Pvt. Ltd.
B 1/I 1 Mohan Cooperative Industrial Area
Mathura Road, New Delhi 110 044
India

SAGE Publications Asia-Pacific Pte. Ltd.
3 Church Street
#10-04 Samsung Hub
Singapore 049483

Printed in the United States of America.

Library of Congress Cataloging-in-Publication Data

Plano Clark, Vicki L.
Mixed methods research : a guide to the field /
Vicki L. Plano Clark, Nataliya V. Ivankova.

pages cm. — (Sage mixed methods research series)
Includes bibliographical references and index.

ISBN 978-1-4833-0675-9 (pbk. : alk. paper)

1. Social sciences—Research—Methodology.
2. Research—Methodology. I. Ivankova, Nataliya V. II. Title.

H62.P564 2016
001.4'2—dc23   2015013704

This book is printed on acid-free paper.

Acquisitions Editor: Vicki Knight
Editorial Assistant: Yvonne McDuffee
Production Editor: Veronica Stapleton Hooper
Copy Editor: Megan Markanich
Typesetter: Hurix Systems Private Ltd.
Proofreader: Jennifer Grubba
Indexer: Sheila Bodell
Cover Designer: Anupama Krishnan
Marketing Manager: Nicole Elliott

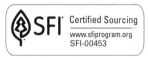
SFI® Certified Sourcing
www.sfiprogram.org
SFI-00453

15 16 17 18 19 10 9 8 7 6 5 4 3 2 1

BRIEF CONTENTS

DETAILED CONTENTS

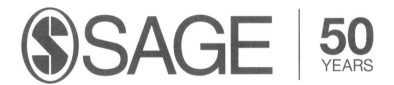

SAGE was founded in 1965 by Sara Miller McCune to support the dissemination of usable knowledge by publishing innovative and high-quality research and teaching content. Today, we publish more than 850 journals, including those of more than 300 learned societies, more than 800 new books per year, and a growing range of library products including archives, data, case studies, reports, and video. SAGE remains majority-owned by our founder, and after Sara's lifetime will become owned by a charitable trust that secures our continued independence.

Los Angeles | London | New Delhi | Singapore | Washington DC

LIST OF FIGURES, TABLES, AND BOXES

Figures

Boxes

PREFACE

WELCOME AND PURPOSE

Welcome to the field of mixed methods research! This field has emerged as a formalized field since the late 1980s from scholars' collective efforts to understand the process of mixing quantitative and qualitative methods to better understand research problems. Scholars have brought different approaches to understanding mixed methods research, such as trying to understand it philosophically, methodologically, theoretically, and even logistically. Scholars have also approached mixed methods research from many different contexts including a wide range of disciplines and nationalities. Supported by the many perspectives, researchers have shown increasing acceptance of mixed methods research, and its use in research practice continues to grow in prevalence and sophistication.

With all of these developments, it is a good time to learn about mixed methods research. However, for those who are new to mixed methods research, it can also be challenging to navigate the mixed methods field and understand the different perspectives, nuances, and debates about mixed methods that are taking place in the mixed methods literature. Throughout our work teaching graduate courses about mixed methods research, offering workshops on mixed methods, and consulting researchers in using mixed methods research, we have found that there is a need for a user-friendly book that introduces students, researchers, and scholars to the dynamic field of mixed methods research. This book is our attempt to address this need.

This book takes a different approach from other books about mixed methods research that focus more on planning and implementing a mixed methods study and all the necessary details in that process. The purpose of this book is to serve as a guide to the field of mixed methods by providing an accessible introduction to mixed methods research that highlights the major topics, perspectives, and ongoing debates in the field and addresses how these topics relate to and shape the practice of mixed methods research. We advance a socio-ecological conceptual framework for the field of mixed methods research that we developed to help the readers understand the importance of these relationships and influences on the mixed methods research process that forms the core of mixed methods research practice. Therefore, this book first introduces readers to the basics of the mixed methods research process and then unravels the influences of multiple methodological content considerations and research contexts that shape the mixed methods research process and are of major concern in the field of mixed methods research.

OVERVIEW OF THE BOOK

We have organized the structure of this book using our socio-ecological conceptual framework for the field of mixed methods research. Part I of the book (Chapters 1 and 2) opens with a discussion of the essence of mixed methods research, an introduction to the field of mixed methods research and our conceptual framework for describing the field, and a discussion of the mixed methods research process that is at the core of the practice of mixed methods research. Part II (Chapters 3–7) then focuses on the important methodological content considerations that directly influence the mixed methods research process: what mixed methods research is, why it is used, how it is designed, how it intersects with other approaches, and how it is assessed. Part III (Chapters 8–10) describes the major contexts that shape mixed methods research practice, which we discuss as personal, interpersonal, and social contexts and examines important topics such as philosophical assumptions, research ethics, and disciplinary conventions. The book concludes in Part IV (Chapter 11) with reflections about the future of the field and its implications for different types of mixed methods research practice.

PEDAGOGICAL FEATURES

The aim of this book is to provide readers with a guide to the field of mixed methods research. Just as a travel guide aims to introduce the landscape, customs, and attractions of a location, this guide to the field of mixed methods research aims to introduce the major topics, perspectives, and issues of mixed methods research. We have included several pedagogical elements that facilitate this "guidebook" approach.

We begin the book by introducing our *socio-ecological framework for mixed methods research* in Chapter 1. This conceptual framework identifies the major topics addressed in the field of mixed methods research and describes how these topics relate to the mixed methods research process. The organization of the chapters is based on this conceptual framework and reflects many of the questions that scholars new to mixed methods research have about this approach. Within each chapter, we present the content by introducing the major perspectives that exist in the field about the topic; providing examples from the mixed methods literature and mixed methods studies; identifying issues and debates found in the field; and considering implications for mixed methods research practice including reading about, reviewing, and conducting mixed methods research.

We start each chapter by outlining the learning objectives and providing a list of key concepts. The *learning objectives* have a practical focus by identifying what the reader should be able to do after completing the chapter, and we revisit the learning objectives at the end of the chapter to organize our summary comments. The *key concepts* are the important terms and associated definitions that will be introduced in the chapter. The terms are ordered to match the flow of the content in the chapter so that they provide an advanced organizer of the information in addition to a chapter glossary. We bold each of the key terms when it is discussed within the chapter to highlight its importance for understanding the chapter content.

We conclude each chapter by offering advice and providing application questions and key resources. Each chapter includes a box feature that lists our advice for applying the chapter content to readers' mixed methods research practice. The application questions prompt readers to apply the chapter content to their own mixed methods research situations and encourage them to grapple with the complexities of the mixed methods field. The key resources provide our recommendations for scholarly publications that readers should examine for further information and different perspectives about the chapter content. Select key resources are also available to readers through the book's website (http://study.sagepub.com/planoclark) for further examination of the chapter topics.

AUDIENCES FOR THE BOOK

This book aims to appeal to anyone wanting an introduction to the field of mixed methods research. This book is intended for those who are interested in applying mixed methods research in their own studies *and* for those who want to be informed consumers and reviewers of mixed methods research. The primary audiences for the book include students and researchers considering a mixed methods approach and who are interested in learning about and potentially applying mixed methods research. This book can be used as a primary or supplemental text in graduate and upper-level undergraduate mixed methods courses or research methods courses that incorporate mixed methods. This book does not assume that the reader is actively planning or conducting a mixed methods study.

Having a basic understanding of the field of mixed methods research is important for all stakeholders who are involved in advocating for, learning about, teaching, planning, conducting, disseminating, and reviewing mixed methods research. Therefore, secondary audiences for the book include reviewers of proposals for funding, journal editors, and reviewers of manuscripts charged with assessing the rigor and quality of proposed or completed mixed methods studies. The book may also be of interest to professionals engaged in community-based participatory research (CBPR) projects who seek to enhance their research by including mixed methods and policy makers who make decisions about priorities for funding and policies for academic programs.

CONNECTION TO THE SAGE
MIXED METHODS RESEARCH SERIES

We are pleased to complete this book both as authors and particularly as the editors of the SAGE Mixed Methods Research Series. Our goals for the Series include developing books that offer practical guidance to readers, highlight essential aspects of mixed methods research, and provide a venue that will continue to evolve and grow as the frontiers of the field of mixed methods research continue to expand. This book aims to help meet these goals in two primary ways. First, as the third volume of the Series, we believe it offers a new approach for describing the field and offering practical insights for how readers can negotiate the considerations and influences involved in mixed methods research practice. In particular, it highlights the important role that different contexts play in mixed methods research. Second, this book also sheds light on how we, as editors, view the field of mixed methods research. It describes our overarching perspective for the range of topics we find important to the field of mixed methods research and exemplifies our interest in works that cut across multiple topics, contexts, and disciplines to examine the dynamic interactions and relationships that occur among topics.

There is currently much enthusiasm and excitement for the use of mixed methods research as a rigorous and effective means for addressing many of the research problems of interest today. We hope that this book, along with all the other volumes of the SAGE Mixed Methods Research Series, will provide readers with the practical knowledge to not only share in that excitement but to also engage in the ongoing conversations and research practices that make up the field of mixed methods research. Welcome to all that the field of mixed methods research has to offer!

ACKNOWLEDGMENTS

Our work on this book, and the SAGE Mixed Methods Research Series more generally, is the culmination of our collective experiences within the field of mixed methods research over the past 15 years. Throughout this time, there are many individuals who have helped to advance our thinking about and opportunities for applying mixed methods research, and we gratefully acknowledge their support.

First and foremost, we are thankful for the extensive support and encouragement we have both received from our respective programs, departments, and schools at the University of Cincinnati and University of Alabama at Birmingham. We have benefitted greatly from the opportunity to teach multiple courses on mixed methods research, to present our ideas in workshops and conferences, to discuss our framework with colleagues, and to receive valuable feedback throughout these opportunities.

We also are indebted to the students who enrolled in our Mixed Methods Research I courses during the development of this book. Their insightful questions, innovative applications, and passion for mixed methods regularly advanced our own thinking about mixed methods and the field of mixed methods research. We thank each and every one of you: Tolu Aduroja, Sally Bethart, Will Brewer, Melinda Butsch-Kovacic, Suguna Chundur, Rachael Clark, Katherine Clarke-Myers, Jennifer Crimiel, Juanita Darden-Jones, Melissa DeJonckheere, Jonathan Engelman, Rimma Foltzer, Lori Foote, Karla Gacasan, L. Nicole Hammons, M. Gail Headley, Tracy Herrmann, Leah Howell, Brenda Jacklitsch, Stacey Janz, Alan Jones, David Jones, Laura Kelley, Jessica Kestler, Jacqueline Knapke, Cassandra Krumpelmann, Joshua Magee, Daniel Marschner, Dennis McCay, Timiya Nolan, William Opoku-Agyeman, Lindsay Owens, Kelly Randall, Khahlia Sanders, Laura Saylor, Jean Scholz, Peggy Shannon-Baker, Marisha Speights, John Stegall, Vicky Stone-Gale, Pamela Theurer, Amy Thompson, Susan Tyler, Janet Walton, Vanessa White, Bryan Wilbanks, and Kenneth Woodson.

We are especially grateful for the guidance that we have received from leaders in the field of mixed methods research. Without question, our work has been most influenced by the writings and mentoring from John W. Creswell at the University of Nebraska–Lincoln. He introduced both of us to the field of mixed methods research as graduate students, supported our development as methodologists through the work of the Office of Qualitative and Mixed Methods Research, and has continued to support our professional growth throughout the years. Several others in the field of mixed methods research have also made important contributions to our thinking about mixed methods through their feedback and supportive interactions. We especially thank Joe Maxwell, Donna Mertens, Abbas Tashakkori, and Charles Teddlie.

None of this work would be possible without the amazing support of family and friends that we have received throughout the years. We are so very thankful for the support of our husbands, Mark and Ivan, who sustained us throughout this book writing process (and everything else). Thank you also to Igor, Ariel, A. J., our moms, and Marilyn Armstrong.

Finally, we thank the professionals who have worked with us throughout this process. We thank Vicki Knight, publisher at SAGE, for her vision to initiate the *Mixed Methods Research Series* and her support and patience as we worked our way through this project. We also thank Yvonne McDuffee, Megan Markanich, and Veronica Stapleton Hooper for their logistical, technical, and editorial assistance. In addition, we are thankful for the invaluable assistance from Katelyn Scott at the University of Cincinnati, the graphic designer who turned our ideas into user-friendly visuals. We are also grateful to several individuals who provided feedback on early drafts of the materials, including Rachael Clark, Ganisher Davlyatov, Khahlia Sanders, Chris Swoboda, and Janet Walton. We appreciate the thoughtful and constructive feedback that we received from our reviewers: Theresa A. Beery, University of Cincinnati; Deborah Gioia, University of Maryland, Baltimore; Michelle C. Howell Smith, University of Nebraska–Lincoln; Tera R. Jordan, Iowa State University; Fairuz J. Lutz, Wesley College; Arturo Olivárez Jr., The University of Texas at El Paso; Elias Ortega-Aponte, Drew University; Mary E. Siegrist, Webster University; Holly Thomas, Carleton University; Daphne C. Watkins, University of Michigan.

ABOUT THE AUTHORS

Vicki L. Plano Clark (Ph.D., University of Nebraska–Lincoln) is an assistant professor in the Quantitative and Mixed Methods Research Methodologies concentration of Educational Studies at the University of Cincinnati (UC). Her teaching focuses on foundations of research methodologies and mixed methods research, including a two-semester mixed methods sequence and special topics courses. As a methodologist specializing in mixed methods research, her scholarship aims to delineate useful designs for conducting mixed methods research, examine procedural issues associated with these designs, and consider larger questions about the contexts for the adoption and use of mixed methods. She has also coauthored several books with John W. Creswell, including *Designing and Conducting Mixed Methods Research* (2007, 2011; SAGE), *The Mixed Methods Reader* (2008; SAGE), and *Understanding Research: A Consumer's Guide* (2010, 2015; Pearson Education). She was the founding managing editor for the *Journal of Mixed Methods Research* (JMMR) and currently serves as an associate editor. In 2011, she co-led the development of *Best Practices for Mixed Methods in the Health Sciences* for the National Institutes of Health (NIH) Office of Behavioral and Social Sciences Research. She is a founding coeditor of the SAGE Mixed Methods Research Series.

As an applied research methodologist, Vicki also engages in research and evaluation projects on a wide array of topics such as the management of cancer pain, the identity development of STEM graduate students, the professional development of teachers of Chinese, and the effectiveness of school reform initiatives. Before joining UC, she was the director of the Office of Qualitative and Mixed Methods Research, a service and research unit that provides methodological support for proposal development and funded projects at the University of Nebraska–Lincoln. Originally trained in physics, she spent 12 years developing innovative curricular materials for introductory physics as the physics laboratory manager at the University of Nebraska–Lincoln.

Nataliya V. Ivankova (Ph.D., University of Nebraska–Lincoln; M.P.H., University of Alabama at Birmingham [UAB]) holds a dual appointment as associate professor in the Department of Health Services Administration (School of Health Professions) and the Department of Acute, Chronic and Continuing Care (School of Nursing) at UAB. She teaches graduate research methods courses, including Philosophy of Science, a two-semester sequence in mixed methods research, mixed methods applications in community-based action research, and advanced courses in qualitative research design. Her expertise is in qualitative inquiry and mixed methods research and their applications across disciplines. Her long-standing interest is in the use of mixed methods in community-based participatory action research, implementation science, and translational research, which resulted in the book *Mixed Methods Applications in Action Research: From Methods to Community Action* (2015; SAGE).

In addition to teaching, Nataliya mentors doctoral students in their dissertation research, and postdoctoral fellows and junior faculty in their qualitative and mixed methods funded research projects. She serves as consultant, coinvestigator, and methodologist on externally and internally funded projects in education, health care management, nursing, and public health. She is a founding coeditor of the SAGE Mixed Methods Research Series and serves as associate editor for the *Journal of Mixed Methods Research* (JMMR) and qualitative research editor for the *American Journal of Health Behavior*. For several years, she chaired the Special Interest Group *Mixed Methods Research* within the American Educational Research Association. Currently, she is actively involved with the Mixed Methods International Research Association (MMIRA) as chair of the Communication & Marketing Committee. Prior to coming to UAB, Nataliya was research projects coordinator in the Office of Qualitative and Mixed Methods Research at the University of Nebraska–Lincoln. During the first eighteen years of her professional career, she served as a member of the faculty and also as dean for admissions at the Izmail State University in Ukraine.

To our mothers Ellen Plano and Tamara Ivankova
Two amazing women who continue to support and inspire us both

PART I

A CONCEPTUAL FRAMEWORK FOR THE FIELD OF MIXED METHODS RESEARCH

Welcome to the field of mixed methods research! We begin this book by considering the expanding field of mixed methods research and how it is becoming increasingly complex for scholars like you to navigate it. We explain the need for a conceptual framework that can serve as a guide to understanding the complexity of the field and introduce our socio-ecological framework for the field of mixed methods research. This framework forms the core of this book and guides our discussions about how different methodological considerations and contexts shape the process of mixed methods research that underlies mixed methods research practice. In the chapters that follow in Part I, we first describe our framework and illustrate its use to understanding mixed methods research practice. We then begin the discussion of the components of our framework by describing the mixed methods research process, which forms the centerpiece of the framework. The two chapters in Part I are as follows:

Chapter 1: Why a Guide to the Field of Mixed Methods Research? Introducing a Conceptual Framework of the Field

Chapter 2: What Is the Core of Mixed Methods Research Practice? Introducing the Mixed Methods Research Process

⚜ ONE ⚜

WHY A GUIDE TO THE FIELD OF MIXED METHODS RESEARCH?

INTRODUCING A CONCEPTUAL FRAMEWORK OF THE FIELD

What is mixed methods research? You have probably heard or seen these words when reading research studies or scanning conference abstracts in your area of interest. It is not surprising as mixed methods research is becoming more popular and accepted across disciplines and countries. However, the expansion and growth of mixed methods research has also triggered the emergence of different views and perspectives about mixed methods, which makes the field of mixed methods more complex and difficult to navigate for researchers who are new to this approach. Being able to understand the issues, controversies, and debates about mixed methods and how they influence the different ways scholars apply mixed methods in their research practice is essential to successfully apply mixed methods to your research interests. Therefore, in this opening chapter, we provide an overview of the field of mixed methods research and introduce our socio-ecological framework that can serve as a guide to understanding the field in a practical and applied way. This conceptual framework also foreshadows our discussion of mixed methods research in the rest of the chapters in this book.

LEARNING OBJECTIVES

This chapter aims to provide a brief overview of the field of mixed methods research and introduce the socio-ecological framework for mixed methods research so you are able to do the following:

- Describe the essence of the mixed methods approach to research and its fundamental principle.

3

- Understand the expansion of the field of mixed methods research and its related controversies and issues.
- Consider the socio-ecological framework for mixed methods research as a guide to the field.

CHAPTER 1 KEY CONCEPTS

The following key concepts will help you navigate through the main considerations related to understanding the field of mixed methods research as they are introduced in the chapter:

- **Mixed methods research:** A process of research in which researchers integrate quantitative and qualitative methods of data collection and analysis to best understand a research purpose. The way this process unfolds in a given study is shaped by mixed methods research content considerations and researchers' personal, interpersonal, and social contexts.
- **Fundamental principle of mixed methods research:** The belief that research methods should be integrated or mixed building on their complementary strengths and nonoverlapping weaknesses.
- **Integration or mixing:** An explicit interrelating of the quantitative and qualitative components within a study.
- **Quantitative research:** A research approach that examines the relationships between variables by collecting and analyzing numeric data expressed in numbers or scores.
- **Qualitative research:** A research approach that focuses on exploring individuals' experiences with a phenomenon by collecting and analyzing narrative or text data expressed in words and images.
- **Field of mixed methods research:** The body of literature and community of scholars that discusses and applies all aspects of mixed methods research.
- **Mixed methods research practice:** Any application of mixed methods research in advocating for, planning, conducting, disseminating, and evaluating the mixed methods research approach by researchers, scholars, and other stakeholders.
- **Socio-ecological model:** A conceptual framework that explains the dynamic interrelations that exist among various individual and

environmental factors and forms the basis for our conceptual framework for the field of mixed methods research.

- **Mixed methods research process:** A process of research that underlies a mixed methods research practice and that consists of a research purpose and questions, methods, and inferences.

- **Mixed methods research content:** Methodological considerations that directly inform the mixed methods research process such as how mixed methods is defined, the rationales for its use, the logic of mixed methods designs, how it combines with other methodological approaches and frameworks, and how quality of a mixed methods study is assessed.

- **Mixed methods research contexts:** The circumstances, including beliefs, background, environment, framework, setting, relationships, and research communities, that shape the practice of mixed methods research and in terms of which it can be fully understood and assessed.

THE ESSENCE OF MIXED METHODS RESEARCH

We begin with the discussion of the essence of mixed methods research to help you understand how it differs from other research approaches with which you may be familiar, such as quantitative research and qualitative research. We use two research scenarios to support this discussion and to illustrate the application of mixed methods research. Suppose you want to explore the experiences of learning science for African American girls from low socioeconomic status (SES) communities, or suppose you want to know how people make choices about what colorectal cancer screening method to use. To address these two scenarios, you could employ quantitative research methods such as surveys and identify the relationship between the key variables (e.g., low SES and girls' attitudes to science, or the relationship between a person's gender and race and the preferred method of screening). Alternatively, you could apply qualitative research methods and conduct individual interviews with a few low SES girls to learn about their experiences and needs with learning science or have focus group discussions with groups of individuals to explore the role of different factors in influencing people's decisions in choosing a colorectal cancer screening method. In each of these scenarios, you could consider conducting either a quantitative or a qualitative study to address specific research questions.

Instead of addressing these scenarios separately using a single research approach, you could instead apply the **mixed methods research** approach and integrate or mix quantitative and qualitative methods of data collection and analysis to address the research problem more fully and to obtain the answers to both quantitative and qualitative questions within a single study. Moreover, integrating quantitative and qualitative methods may help you reach more justifiable and more complete study conclusions than using quantitative or qualitative methods alone (Greene & Caracelli, 1997b). To better illustrate this point, we next consider two studies that used mixed methods research to address the discussed research situations.

Box 1.1 presents the abstract of Buck, Cook, Quigley, Eastwood, and Lucas's (2009) mixed methods study that explored the attitudes about learning science of African American girls from low SES communities. The researchers first collected quantitative data from the Modified Attitudes toward Science Inventory to create the attitudes-toward-science profiles of 89 girls based on their attitudes-toward-science scores. The profile information gleaned from this first quantitative phase was explored further in a second qualitative phase during which the researchers interviewed 30 girls from different profiles "to better understand and explain the reasons for the differences in profiles" (p. 391). Thus, addressing the problem in a sequential manner helped the researchers use "qualitative results to assist in explaining and interpreting quantitative findings" (p. 392).

Box 1.1

Abstract of Buck et al.'s (2009) Mixed Methods Study of Low Socioeconomic Status African American Girls' Attitudes to Learning Science

Abstract

The purpose of this study was to increase the science education community's understanding of the experiences and needs of girls who cross the traditional categorical boundaries of gender, race and socioeconomic status in a manner that has left their needs and experience largely invisible. A first of several in a series, this study sought to explore how African American girls from low SES communities position themselves in science learning. We followed a mixed methods sequential explanatory strategy, in which two data collection phases, qualitative following the quantitative, were employed to investigate 89 African-American girls' personal orientations towards science learning. By using quantitative data from the Modified Attitudes toward Science Inventory to organize students into attitude profiles and then sequentially integrating the profile scores with year-long interview data, we found that the girls' orientations towards science were best described in terms of definitions of science, importance of science, experiences with science, and success in science. Therefore, our mixed method analysis provided four personality orientations which linked success in school and experiences with science to confidence and importance of science and definitions of science to value/desire. In our efforts to decrease the achievement gap, we concluded there should be more emphasis on conceptual understanding and problem-solving skills, while still being cognizant of the danger of losing the connection between science and society which so often plagues achievement focused efforts. Our continued efforts with this group of girls will center on these instructional techniques with the goal of addressing the needs of all science learners.

Source: Buck, G., Cook, K., Quigley, C., Eastwood, J., & Lucas, Y. (2009). Profiles of urban, low SES, African American girls' attitudes toward science: A sequential explanatory mixed methods study. *Journal of Mixed Methods Research, 3*(4), 386–410.

Now consider the abstract of a mixed methods study of factors influencing choices for colorectal cancer screening conducted by Ruffin, Creswell, Jimbo, and Fetters (2009) and presented in Box 1.2. In this study, the researchers simultaneously collected and analyzed quantitative survey data and qualitative focus group data from 93 individuals who were 50 years of age or older and reported not having been screened for colorectal cancer in the past 10 years. The researchers interpreted the two sets of quantitative and qualitative results together because by integrating the results "a more robust and complete understanding is possible [rather] than the use of either data source alone" (p. 80).

Box 1.2

Abstract of Ruffin et al.'s (2009) Mixed Methods Study of Factors Influencing Choices for Colorectal Cancer Screening

Abstract

We investigated factors that influence choice of colorectal cancer (CRC) screening test and assessed the most- and least-preferred options among fecal occult blood testing (FOBT), flexible sigmoidoscopy, colonoscopy, and double contrast barium enema among adults with varied race, gender, and geographic region demographics. Mixed methods data collection consisted of 10 focus group interviews and a survey of the 93 focus group participants.

Participants were ≥50 years of age and reported not having been screened for colorectal cancer in the last ten years. Analyses examined differences by race, gender, and geographic location. Participants had modest knowledge about CRC and there were fewer correct answers to knowledge questions by African Americans. Participants recognized value of early detection, and identified health symptoms and their doctor's recommendation as influential for obtaining CRC screening. They chose colonoscopy and FOBT as the most preferred tests, while barium enema was least preferred. The analysis revealed intra-group variations in preference, though there were no significant differences by race, gender, or location. Openness of discussing this sensitive topic, lack of knowledge about colorectal cancer and screening costs, and diversity of preferences expressed within study groups suggest the importance of patient-physician dialogue about colorectal cancer screening options. New approaches to promoting colorectal cancer screening need to explore methods to facilitate patients establishing and expressing preferences among the screening options.

Source: Ruffin, M.T., IV, Creswell, J.W., Jimbo, M., & Fetters, M.D. (2009). Factors influencing choices for colorectal cancer screening among previously unscreened African and Caucasian Americans: Findings from a triangulation mixed methods investigation. *Journal of Community Health, 34*(2), 79–89.

As you can see from these two examples of mixed methods studies, by capitalizing on the strengths of each quantitative and qualitative method, researchers can produce stronger and more credible studies that can yield both complementary and corroborating evidence about the research problem of interest. Additionally, integrating quantitative and qualitative methods within one study can help researchers exclude or minimize potential alternative explanations of the results, while at the same time provide enough information to explain the divergent aspects of the studied phenomenon. Johnson and Turner (2003) referred to this advantage of mixed methods as a **fundamental principle of mixed methods research.** In their words, "Methods should be mixed in a way that has complementary strengths and nonoverlapping weaknesses" (p. 299).

Therefore, understanding this fundamental principle of mixed methods research is important for you to understand the essence of the mixed methods approach. As it is clear from Johnson and Turner's (2003) explanation of this principle, the idea of the integration or mixing of quantitative and qualitative methods is central to mixed methods research. **Integration or mixing** is an explicit interrelating of the quantitative and qualitative components within a study. Figure 1.1 presents our conceptual view of mixed methods research that highlights this integration aspect.

Three overlapping spheres symbolize three approaches to research: quantitative, qualitative, and mixed. **Quantitative research** examines the relationships among variables by collecting and analyzing numeric data expressed in numbers or scores using standardized measurement instruments. **Qualitative research** focuses on exploring individuals' experiences with a phenomenon of interest by collecting and analyzing narrative or text data expressed in words and images using broad open-ended questions. Mixed methods research is depicted by several nested, dashed, shaded spheres of different tones and is positioned in the center to capture where the quantitative and qualitative spheres connect or merge with each other. Different dashed shaded spheres represent different degrees of integration of the qualitative and quantitative methods in a mixed methods study, which may vary from study to study depending on the specific research purpose—for example, ranging from a more complete integration shown by the larger, dark shaded sphere to a limited integration reflected by the small, light shaded sphere. The direction of the arrows indicates whether the study is a *mono-method study*—that is, straight quantitative or qualitative (solid horizontal arrows in quantitative and

Figure 1.1   Conceptualization of Mixed Methods Research

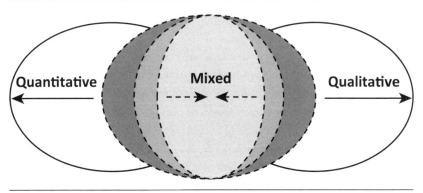

SOURCE: Adapted from Ivankova, N. V. (2015). *Mixed methods applications in action research: From methods to community action* with permission of SAGE Publications, Inc.

qualitative spheres point in opposite directions) or whether the study is a mixed methods study (dashed horizontal arrows point to each other indicating connecting or merging of the quantitative and qualitative spheres).

THE FIELD OF MIXED METHODS RESEARCH

The advantages of mixed methods research for addressing complex study purposes within the boundaries of a single study has led to its acceptance and application across disciplines and countries (Alise & Teddlie, 2010; Creswell, 2010; Ivankova & Kawamura, 2010; Plano Clark, 2010). Building from early writings in the 1970s and 1980s (e.g., Greene, Caracelli, & Graham, 1989; Reichardt & Cook, 1979), the mixed methods approach is now extensively applied in the social, behavioral, and health sciences. The utility, strength, and acceptance of mixed methods is emphasized by its recognition as the third research paradigm (Johnson & Onwuegbuzie, 2004), the third methodological movement (Teddlie & Tashakkori, 2003), the third research community (Teddlie & Tashakkori, 2009), and the third research approach (Creswell, 2014).

The expansion in the use and acceptance of mixed methods has occurred hand in hand with the growth of the **field of mixed methods research.** This field encompasses the body of literature and community of scholars that discusses and applies all aspects of mixed methods research. Signs of the field's growth abound with mixed methods textbooks and reference books, including two editions of the *SAGE Handbook of Mixed Methods in Social & Behavioral Research* (Tashakkori & Teddlie, 2003a, 2010b), *The Oxford Handbook of Multimethod and Mixed Methods Research Inquiry* (Hesse-Biber & Johnson, 2015), numerous empirical and methodological mixed methods articles and reviews, and special peer-reviewed journal issues. Two cross-disciplinary international journals, the *Journal of Mixed Methods Research* (JMMR) and the *International Journal of Multiple Research Approaches,* are exclusively devoted to this research approach.

Professional conferences are also available that offer mixed methods researchers forums for exchanging ideas about mixed methods, including the American Educational Research Association Special Interest Group "Mixed Methods Research," the American Evaluation Association Topical Interest Group "Mixed Methods Evaluation," and the annual International Mixed Methods Conference (first held in 2005). The Mixed Methods International Research Association (MMIRA) was formed in 2013 to promote the development of an international and interdisciplinary mixed methods research community that unites mixed methods researchers around the world (http://www.mmira.org).

The popularity of mixed methods research is also growing among agencies that fund research. In the United States, major funding agencies, such as the National Institutes of Health (NIH), the National Science Foundation, the Department of Education, and the Patient-Centered Outcomes Research Institute are supporting mixed methods projects. For example, the NIH published *Best Practices for Mixed Methods Research in the Health Sciences* (Creswell, Klassen, Plano Clark, & Smith for the Office of Behavioral and Social Sciences Research, 2011) to guide health sciences researchers on how to develop and evaluate scientifically sound proposals for mixed methods funded studies. The Economic and Social Research Council in the United Kingdom also plays a prominent role in funding mixed methods studies through its Research Methods Program.

With the extensive growth, the field of mixed methods is also becoming increasingly complex, nuanced, and specialized (Grbich, 2007; Hesse-Biber & Johnson, 2013; Tashakkori & Creswell, 2007b; Tashakkori & Teddlie, 2010b). Different views and perspectives about mixed methods have emerged that often stem from differences in scholars' philosophical stances and epistemological practices adopted in their disciplines (Teddlie & Tashakkori, 2009). As scholars with different philosophical and disciplinary contexts continue to engage with mixed methods research, they generate important controversies, issues, and debates that call for further discourse and dialogue among the many different perspectives and also for the need to understand how these perspectives shape the field of mixed methods research. This book is our answer to this call for continued dialogue and understanding of the field of mixed methods research.

THE NEED FOR A GUIDE FOR NAVIGATING THE FIELD OF MIXED METHODS RESEARCH

The growth of sophistication within the field of mixed methods and the calls for increased discourse and dialogue are both critically important. All new substantive and methodological fields go through a development process complete with growing pains and many advances. As such, we believe the ongoing expansion of the field of mixed methods research and the accompanying constructive debates about its theoretical, methodological, and practical aspects are a necessary part of its overall development process. This ongoing development process means that mixed methods is "a new field where the terrain is not yet fully formed" and learning about it may be particularly complex (Greene, 2010, p. 2).

While pluralism in perspectives and practices is welcome and is a healthy element in the continued growth of the field, it adds complexity to understanding and navigating the field of mixed methods. Therefore, whenever you, as well as other scholars, engage in mixed methods research practice, you have to consider the multiple perspectives and complexity of the field. We define *mixed methods research practice* as any application of mixed methods research in advocating for, planning, conducting, disseminating, and evaluating the mixed methods research approach by researchers, scholars, and other stakeholders. Mixed methods research practice is a complex and multifaceted endeavor that requires scholars to stay current with the new developments and nuances of the field. If you are new to mixed methods research, you can benefit from a conceptual framework that serves as a guide to the field and provides a concise introduction to mixed methods research and highlights the current trends and controversies in the field. More specifically, a guiding framework can assist you in understanding and navigating the important issues of mixed methods research and help you connect the available theoretical and methodological writings to the practical issues that occur when using mixed methods research. We also believe such a framework can help you better understand the influences of multiple personal, interpersonal, and social contexts that shape how you read, review, evaluate, design, and conduct mixed methods research—that is, how you engage in mixed methods research practice.

That said, we are not the first to emphasize the value of a conceptual framework for examining the field of mixed methods. Mixed methods authors have suggested several frameworks for considering the depth and breadth and limitations of the field of mixed methods research. For example, Greene (2008) proposed a framework of four methodological domains (i.e., philosophy, methodology, practical guidelines, and sociopolitical commitments) to frame the field of mixed methods as a distinctive methodology. Creswell (2009) mapped the field into five domains (philosophical and theoretical issues, techniques of mixed methods, nature of mixed methods, adoption and use of mixed methods, and politicization of mixed methods). Tashakkori and Teddlie (2010b) conceptualized the field of mixed methods in three broad domains (conceptual, methods and methodology, and contemporary applications). Each of these authors acknowledged that their mixed methods research frameworks could include additional domains to represent the field of mixed methods more completely and in more detail.

These and other frameworks present thoughtful examinations of the status of the field of mixed methods research and serve as meaningful bases from which to conceptualize and assess mixed methods as a methodology. Despite the value of the existing frameworks, they also have some limitations. These frameworks tend to emphasize theoretical and methodological discussions about mixed methods research aimed at methodologists and outweigh practical recommendations for how scholars can understand and navigate the field of mixed methods. These frameworks also tend to present the domains as largely disconnected entities with minimal attention to how they may interact within the field or within one particular mixed methods study.

If you are a scholar who is new to mixed methods research, then the complexity of the existing methodologically focused frameworks of the mixed methods field may create additional challenges for learning about this research approach. Moreover, the complexity and sometimes disconnected views that make up several of the existing frameworks may be seen as a barrier if you seek to position yourself within a mixed methods research approach because you may not readily realize the interacting influences of multiple contexts on your mixed methods research practice. Our decision to develop a new conceptual framework grew from our belief that a more comprehensive and practically focused framework that can explain the relationships that influence and shape scholars' mixed methods research practices is needed. Such a framework can be useful by making the dynamic nature of the field of mixed methods research more apparent and understandable and may be viewed as a helpful complement to the more theoretically oriented frameworks that currently exist. Additionally, such a framework can be helpful for considering the existing body of the literature about mixed methods research, interacting with the community of scholars that use mixed methods, and engaging in mixed methods research practices that are part of the field of mixed methods research.

THE SOCIO-ECOLOGICAL FRAMEWORK FOR THE FIELD OF MIXED METHODS RESEARCH

In this section, we introduce our conceptual framework that attempts to explain the system of dynamic complex relationships that exists in the field of mixed methods research and that uniquely shapes scholars' mixed methods research practices. We developed our framework using an ecological systems approach that was informed by the ecological framework for human development advanced by Bronfenbrenner (1979) and socio-ecological perspectives of McLeroy, Bibeau, Steckler, and Glanz (1988), Stokols (1996), and others. We chose the **socio-ecological model** as the basis for our conceptual framework to help understand and explain the field of mixed methods research because this model recognizes and explains the interwoven dynamic relationships that exist between various individual and environmental factors, such as personal, interpersonal, organizational, community, and societal contexts. These factors form different levels within the system of relationships that aims at explaining the person's complex interactions with his or her environment and the contextual nature of such interactions. From the socio-ecological perspective, these relationships shape an individual's beliefs, knowledge, and experiences in multiple unique ways and predetermine how an individual interacts with his or her environment. Likewise, mixed methods research practice is a dynamic and interactive process that involves multiple domains and contexts, and we wanted a framework for describing and understanding the many relationships that occur in this process. In our view, our socio-ecological framework for mixed methods research captures the complexity and nuances of mixed methods and can serve as a guide to navigate and explain the field of mixed methods research.

We depicted our conceptual framework for mixed methods research in Figure 1.2 and described its components in Table 1.1. This framework takes the form of a mixed methods socio-ecological model of interconnected levels and their components consisting of the mixed methods research process, mixed methods research content, and mixed methods research contexts. We place the mixed methods research process at the center of the framework

Figure 1.2 The Socio-Ecological Framework for the Field of Mixed Methods Research

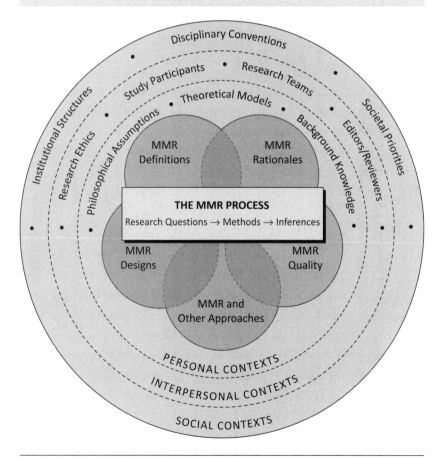

NOTE: MMR = mixed methods research.

Table 1.1 Levels and Components of the Socio-Ecological Framework for the Field of Mixed Methods Research

Major Levels	Level Components	Component Descriptions
Mixed methods research process (central box in Figure 1.2)	The process consisting of research purpose and questions, methods, and inferences	• This component addresses the process of conceptualizing, designing, and conducting mixed methods research in response to a research question using appropriate methods and generating relevant inferences. The mixed methods research process will be discussed further in Chapter 2.
Mixed methods research content (five overlapping inner circles in Figure 1.2)	Mixed methods research definitions	• This component addresses the different perspectives for how mixed methods research is defined. Mixed methods research definitions will be discussed further in Chapter 3.
	Mixed methods research rationales	• This component addresses the different rationales available that provide the argument and reasons for using mixed methods. Mixed methods research rationales will be discussed further in Chapter 4.
	Mixed methods research designs	• This component addresses how to design a mixed methods research study and acknowledges the variety of basic logics for how mixed methods designs are conceptualized. Mixed methods research designs will be discussed further in Chapter 5.
	Mixed methods research and other approaches	• This component addresses different ways for how mixed methods research can intersect with other research designs, methodological approaches, and theoretical frameworks. Mixed methods research intersection with other approaches will be discussed further in Chapter 6.

Mixed methods research quality		• This component addresses how to assess and plan for quality in mixed methods research and acknowledges the variety of perspectives found about quality. Mixed methods research quality will be discussed further in Chapter 7.
Mixed methods research contexts (three nested outer circles in Figure 1.2)	Personal contexts	• This component addresses personal contexts (e.g., philosophical assumptions, theoretical models, and background knowledge) important to mixed methods research and considers how they shape one's mixed methods research content considerations and research practice. Personal contexts for mixed methods research will be discussed further in Chapter 8.
	Interpersonal contexts	• This component addresses interpersonal contexts (e.g., research ethics and researchers' relationships with study participants, teams, and reviewers) important to mixed methods research and considers how they shape one's mixed methods research content considerations and research practice. Interpersonal contexts for mixed methods research will be discussed further in Chapter 9.
	Social contexts	• This component addresses social contexts (e.g., institutional structures, disciplinary conventions, and societal priorities) important to mixed methods research and considers how they shape one's mixed methods research content considerations and research practice. Social contexts for mixed methods research will be discussed further in Chapter 10.

because we believe that it unfolds based on the decisions informed by mixed methods research content and that these decisions are dynamically shaped within a system of hierarchical mixed methods research contexts and relationships that ultimately influence and shape scholars' mixed methods research practice. This framework provides the organizational structure of this book, as noted in the third column of Table 1.1. We briefly introduce each level of our socio-ecological framework for mixed methods research in this chapter and further describe and explain each framework component in the subsequent chapters of this book.

Mixed Methods Research Process

We consider mixed methods research to be a process of research where researchers integrate quantitative and qualitative methods of data collection and analysis to best understand a research purpose (Creswell & Plano Clark, 2011). The **mixed methods research process** consists of the research purpose and questions, methods, and inferences that underlie any mixed methods research practice. We view the mixed methods research process as the innermost level of the framework as depicted in the center box of Figure 1.2. It is informed by mixed methods research content considerations, and it is shaped by internal and external contexts.

Mixed Methods Research Content

We view **mixed methods research content** as directly informing the mixed methods research process and the practice of mixed methods research. The way that mixed methods research process unfolds is shaped by a wide array of methodological considerations that we conceptualize as mixed methods research content domains represented by five overlapping inner circles in Figure 1.2. These methodological domains include major decisions that scholars make when they engage in mixed methods research practice, such as how mixed methods is defined, the rationales for its use, the logic of mixed methods designs, how the study design intersects with other methodological approaches and frameworks, and how quality of a mixed methods study is assessed. The methodological considerations are themselves shaped by internal and external contexts.

Mixed Methods Research Contexts

We view mixed methods research contexts as the outermost level of our framework represented by three outer nested circles in Figure 1.2. The way that scholars understand and apply mixed methods research content in their mixed methods research practice is shaped by their personal, interpersonal, and social contexts. **Mixed methods research contexts** include the circumstances, consisting of beliefs, background, environment, framework, setting, relationships, and communities, that shape the practice of mixed methods research and in terms of which it can be fully understood and assessed. These contexts also interact with each other and jointly influence the variety of perspectives found within the methodological considerations and shape how they inform the decisions about the mixed methods research process.

APPLICATION OF THE SOCIO-ECOLOGICAL FRAMEWORK TO A MIXED METHODS STUDY

To illustrate the use of the socio-ecological framework for mixed methods research and to better understand how external and internal factors influence the decisions scholars make about their mixed methods research practice, we provide two examples of the framework application. First, we apply the framework to Ruffin and colleagues' (2009) study that we discussed in this chapter to illustrate how you can use the framework as a scholar when reading and evaluating a published mixed methods study. Next, we apply the framework to one of our own research efforts (Ivankova, 2014) to illustrate how you can use the framework as a researcher when you conceptualize, design, conduct, and disseminate a mixed methods study.

An Example of Applying the Framework to Ruffin et al.'s (2009) Study

Ruffin and colleagues (2009) reported a mixed methods study of factors influencing choices for colorectal cancer screening (see the study abstract in Box 1.2). We applied our framework as we read this study to identify the major components of the study's mixed methods research process, content, and contexts as discussed in the article. Figure 1.3 provides an overview of this mixed methods study as represented by our conceptual framework.

Figure 1.3   Application of the Socio-Ecological Framework for Describing the Mixed Methods Research Process, Content Considerations, and Contexts for Ruffin et al.'s (2009) Study

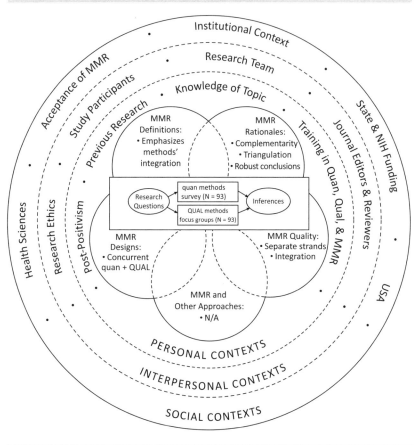

NOTE: MMR = mixed methods research; NIH = National Institutes of Health.

The Mixed Methods Research Process

The study's mixed methods research process is depicted in the center of Figure 1.3. The research team designed this study to quantitatively test for participants' knowledge and beliefs of colorectal cancer and to qualitatively explore the reasons to be screened and the choice of a screening test. Uppercase letters indicate the overall importance of the qualitative method for addressing the study's purpose. The researchers gathered numeric data by surveying the participants during the focus groups before conducting in-depth qualitative discussions. The research team analyzed the quantitative data using statistical procedures and the qualitative data using text analysis procedures. The team combined and interpreted the quantitative and qualitative results to generate integrated study conclusions about the complex factors that ultimately influence the decisions that individuals make about colorectal cancer screening.

The Mixed Methods Research Content

The mixed methods research content considerations that informed this study's research process are summarized in the five overlapping inner circles of Figure 1.3. The study was built from a definition of mixed methods that emphasized integration of quantitative and qualitative data collection and analysis methods and a rationale that these two methods should be triangulated to achieve a more robust and complete understanding of the research issue. The study's approach was informed by the logic for combining the methods in a concurrent (quan + QUAL) mixed methods design. It does not seem that the researchers intersected their mixed methods design with any other methodological approach. The researchers designed the study to be high quality by considering traditional standards for analyzing quantitative and qualitative data and quality in terms of integrating the separate results to generate new insights.

The Mixed Methods Research Contexts

The outer circles in Figure 1.3 indicate the many interrelated contexts that we noted as having influenced the researchers' decisions related to the design and conduct of this mixed methods study. For example, personal contexts included the researchers' postpositivist views on generating knowledge, which guided decisions about the study's variables and the focus of qualitative questions based on previous research. Interpersonal contexts included the interactions that occurred among team members with different roles and training throughout the study and the considerations needed when seeking the University of Michigan Institutional Review Board (IRB) approval for a study on a sensitive health-related issue and in terms of ethical obligations to study participants. The team also had to consider the requirements and the editors' and reviewers' feedback prior to publishing their study in the *Journal of Community Health.* Social contexts included designing and reporting the study's parameters to fit within relevant institutional contexts and align with funding priorities and disciplinary norms in the health sciences.

An Example of Applying the Framework to Ivankova's (2014) Study

As a second example, we apply our conceptual framework to describe one researcher's perspective about how she designed and conducted a mixed methods study that explored how master's and doctoral students engage in learning applied research methods online and what teaching strategies they perceive as being effective (Ivankova, 2014). Figure 1.4 provides an overview of this mixed methods study as represented by our conceptual framework.

Figure 1.4 Application of the Socio-Ecological Framework for Describing the Mixed Methods Research Process, Content Considerations, and Contexts for Ivankova's (2014) Study

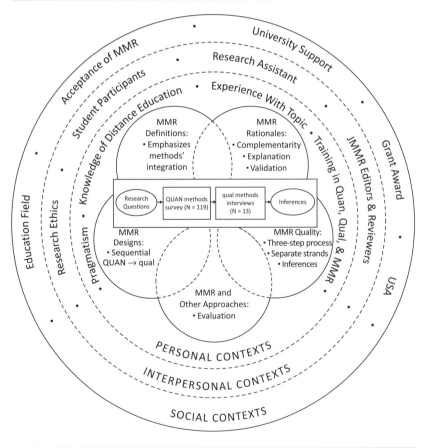

NOTE: JMMR = *Journal of Mixed Methods Research;* MMR = mixed methods research.

The Mixed Methods Research Process

The study's mixed methods research process is depicted in the center of Figure 1.4. Ivankova designed the study to explore the research problem in two sequential quantitative and qualitative phases. Uppercase letters indicate the overall importance of the quantitative method for addressing the study's purpose. First, Ivankova used a survey to collect quantitative data from 119 students who successfully completed at least one online research methods course from a major university in the southeastern United States. She analyzed this information to gain a general description of how students engage in learning applied research methods online and to statistically identify important strategies that enhanced their learning. Then Ivankova conducted qualitative follow-up interviews with 13 purposefully selected survey respondents to seek an explanation of the quantitative results. At the end of the study, she interpreted the quantitative survey and qualitative interview results together to create integrated study conclusions for the posed research questions.

The Mixed Methods Research Content

Five overlapping inner circles of Figure 1.4 represent the mixed methods research content considerations that helped shape the research process during the design and implementation of the study. Ivankova adopted a definition of mixed methods research that emphasized the integration of quantitative and qualitative data and results to draw inferences about a research problem (Tashakkori & Creswell, 2007b). Her rationale for using mixed methods was to explore the research problem by complementing quantitative and qualitative methods to gain a deeper insight into the issue and to ensure the inferences made were valid. She followed the logic for combining the quantitative and qualitative methods in a sequential (QUAN $\rightarrow$ qual) mixed methods design that matched the study purpose of first obtaining a general picture of students' engagement in learning applied research methods online and then elaborating on select quantitative results in more depth using qualitative methods. The study design was also informed by the evaluation approach used in education that employs various data collection and analysis methods to assess students' learning outcomes. Ivankova used a three-step process to ensure the study's quality by first separately assessing the quality of the quantitative and qualitative data and results and next by assessing the credibility of the inferences generated based on the joint interpretation of the survey and interview findings.

The Mixed Methods Research Contexts

The outer circles in Figure 1.4 indicate the interrelated contexts that influenced the design and conduct of this mixed methods study. Personal contexts included Ivankova's long-standing interest in the topic of distance education, her philosophical beliefs of pragmatism that emphasizes the practical value of combining different methods, and her extensive training in and experience with mixed methods research. At the interpersonal level, Ivankova had to obtain approval for conducting a sequential mixed methods study from the university's ethical review board, develop trustworthy and ethical relationships with student–participants and the research assistant, and to comply with the journal guidelines and the editors' and reviewers' feedback when preparing the study manuscript for publication. The influence of social contexts was evident through the adoption of mixed methods in educational research, acceptance of mixed methods at her university, and the internal grant awarded for the study.

USING THE SOCIO-ECOLOGICAL FRAMEWORK TO GUIDE THIS BOOK

As the two examples illustrated, there are many considerations and contexts that inform and shape the design, implementation, and reporting of any mixed methods study. The mixed methods research process, content, and contexts encompass the broad range of topics and diverse perspectives that make up the field of mixed methods research. Approaching the field of mixed methods research from a comprehensive socio-ecological perspective provides an organizational framework for thinking about the field when you read and apply the available literature about mixed methods to your mixed methods research practice. In Chapter 2, we will discuss the mixed methods research process, which is at the core of all mixed methods research practice and is the centerpiece of our framework. From there, we will examine each of the mixed methods research content domains discussed in the field in Part II, and we will explore the contexts that shape the mixed methods research practice in Part III. We conclude the book by considering how these different levels dynamically interact within mixed methods research practice and will continue to encourage the field of mixed methods research to evolve and expand over time.

CONCLUDING COMMENTS

We conclude the chapter by offering some final summary comments organized by the learning objectives stated at the beginning of the chapter.

- **Describe the essence of the mixed methods approach to research and its fundamental principle.** The idea of the integration or mixing of quantitative and qualitative methods is central to mixed methods research. It underscores a fundamental principle of mixed methods research that implies that by capitalizing on the strengths of each quantitative and qualitative method, researchers can produce much stronger and more credible studies. Understanding the essence of mixed methods research is essential for critically reviewing and applying mixed methods research in practice.

- **Understand the expansion of the field of mixed methods research and its related controversies and issues.** Mixed methods research is growing in acceptance and application across disciplines and countries, but it is also becoming increasingly complex, nuanced, and specialized. While pluralism in perspectives and research practices is welcome, it adds complexity to understanding and navigating the field of mixed methods. A framework that serves as a guide to the many topics and perspectives found within the field may assist scholars in learning about the basic issues and practices of mixed methods research.

- **Consider the socio-ecological framework for mixed methods research as a guide to the field.** Our socio-ecological framework for the field of mixed methods research complements existing methodological frameworks and provides a model for understanding the field and how the mixed methods research content and contexts are interrelated and shape scholars' mixed methods research process and practice. Because this framework recognizes the multiple perspectives and nuances within the field of mixed methods research and captures the dynamics and debates of the field, it assists with understanding how to apply the existing body of knowledge about mixed methods to one's research practice.

APPLICATION QUESTIONS

1. Read the mixed methods study abstracts presented in Box 1.1 (Buck et al., 2009) and Box 1.2 (Ruffin et al., 2009). Reflect on what makes these studies mixed methods studies and how the authors applied quantitative and qualitative methods. What differences do you see in how the quantitative and qualitative data collection and analysis were carried out in these two studies? How were the quantitative and qualitative methods integrated?

2. Reflect on the growth of the field of mixed methods research. Why do you think mixed methods research has become so accepted across disciplines and countries?

3. Conduct a quick search of the library databases for mixed methods empirical studies in your discipline. Use the key term *mixed methods* and the name of your discipline. Record the number of mixed methods studies found for each year of publication. What trends do you see in the use of mixed methods research in your discipline across the years?

4. Consider different possible mixed methods research practices (e.g., advocating for, planning, conducting, disseminating, evaluating, and teaching about mixed methods research). Identify three different ways that you might engage in a mixed methods research practice. For each research practice, identify the component(s) of the field of mixed methods research as depicted in our socio-ecological framework that you expect to be particularly important for that practice. Explain why you selected the particular component(s).

5. Read the full study report by Buck et al. (2009), which is available to download as one of the Key Resources noted below. Identify information about the mixed methods research process, content considerations, and contexts that you find in the full article. Based on the socio-ecological framework and the examples found in Figure 1.3 and Figure 1.4,

use the template provided in Figure 1.5 to depict the authors' use of mixed methods research within this study.

6. Locate and read a mixed methods study in your area of interest. Identify information about the mixed methods research process, content considerations, and contexts that you find in the article. Based on the socio-ecological framework and the examples found in Figure 1.3 and Figure 1.4, use the template provided in Figure 1.6 to depict the authors' use of mixed methods research within this study.

Figure 1.5 Application of the Socio-Ecological Framework for Describing the Mixed Methods Research Process, Content Considerations, and Contexts for Buck et al.'s (2009) Study

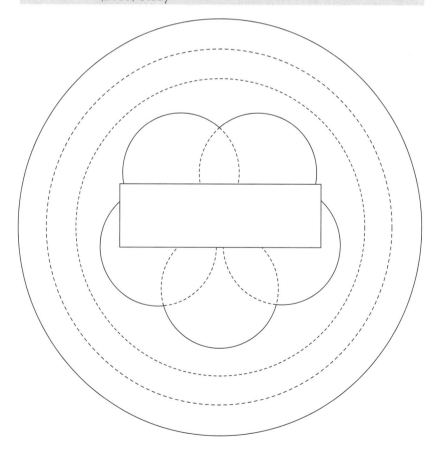

Figure 1.6   Application of the Socio-Ecological Framework for Describing the Mixed Methods Research Process, Content Considerations, and Contexts for a Mixed Methods Study in Your Area of Interest

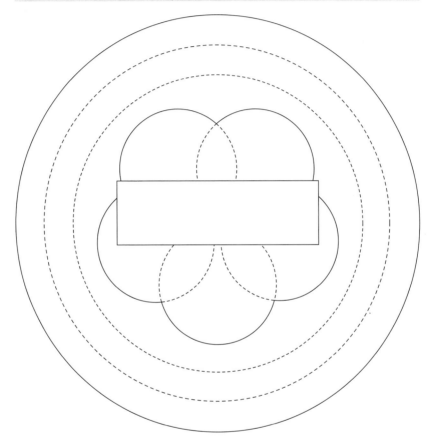

KEY RESOURCES

To learn more about the ongoing development of the field of mixed methods research, we suggest you start with the following resources:

   *1. Johnson, R. B., & Onwuegbuzie, A. (2004). Mixed methods research: A research paradigm whose time has come. *Educational Researcher, 33*(7), 14–26.

- In this article, Johnson and Onwuegbuzie reviewed the historical development of the field of mixed methods. They positioned mixed methods research as the third research paradigm and discussed its essential methodological characteristics.

2. **Creswell, J. W. (2010). Mapping the developing landscape of mixed methods research. In A. Tashakkori & C. Teddlie (Eds.),** *SAGE handbook of mixed methods in social & behavioral research* **(2nd ed., pp. 45–68). Thousand Oaks, CA: Sage.**

- In this book chapter, Creswell provided an overview of the field of mixed methods research and offered varied perspectives on the essence of mixed methods.

*3. **Hesse-Biber, S., & Johnson, R. B. (2013). Coming at things differently: Future directions of possible engagement with mixed methods research [Editorial].** *Journal of Mixed Methods Research,* **7(2), 103–109.**

- In this editorial, Hesse-Biber and Johnson discussed the diverse approaches that are reflected in the mixed methods research community and outlined the opportunities for a continued dialogue among mixed methods researchers.

*4. **Buck, G., Cook, K., Quigley, C., Eastwood, J., & Lucas, Y. (2009). Profiles of urban, low SES, African American girls' attitudes toward science: A sequential explanatory mixed methods study.** *Journal of Mixed Methods Research, 3*(4), 386–410.

- In this article, Buck and colleagues reported on a sequential mixed methods study that explored the attitudes toward science of urban African American girls from low SES communities.

* The key resource is available at the following website: http://study.sagepub.com/planoclark.

⚜ TWO ⚜

WHAT IS THE CORE OF MIXED METHODS RESEARCH PRACTICE?

INTRODUCING THE MIXED METHODS RESEARCH PROCESS

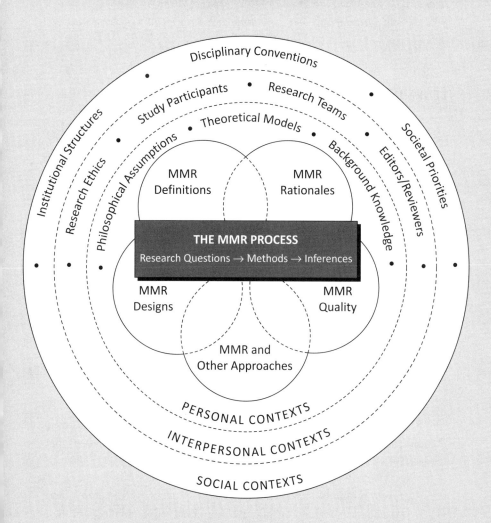

*N*ow that we have introduced the field of mixed methods research and described our socio-ecological framework for navigating the field, you may be wondering how you can apply this framework to your own mixed methods research practice. We recommend starting by examining the mixed methods research process, which is at the core of mixed methods research practice, and looking closely at its basic components. The mixed methods research process forms the centerpiece of our framework. We believe it is important to know the process of mixed methods research to be able to understand how it is informed and shaped by a system of hierarchical contexts and relationships that form the other layers and domains of the framework. Therefore, in this chapter we discuss the mixed methods research process and introduce its major components as well as related issues and debates.

LEARNING OBJECTIVES

This chapter aims to describe the mixed methods research process and its role within the socio-ecological framework for mixed methods research so you are able to do the following:

- Describe the components in the mixed methods research process that is the core of mixed methods research practice.
- Understand the role of the research purpose, objectives, and questions in the mixed methods research process.
- Consider the practical issues related to the use of methods in the mixed methods research process, such as timing, integration, and priority.
- Explain the nature of inferences that are the outcome of the mixed methods research process.

CHAPTER 2 KEY CONCEPTS

The following key concepts will help you navigate through the main considerations related to understanding the mixed methods research process as they are introduced in this chapter:

- **Mixed methods research process:** A process of research where researchers integrate quantitative and qualitative methods of data collection and analysis to best understand a research purpose. It is the core of mixed methods research practice.

- **Research purpose and objectives:** Statements of intent that identify the goals that researchers plan to achieve by undertaking a study.
- **Research questions:** Questions that narrow the research purpose to specific questions that researchers seek to answer in a research study.
- **Timing or sequence:** The temporal relationship between the quantitative and qualitative methods of data collection and analysis in a mixed methods study.
- **Integration or mixing:** An explicit interrelating of the quantitative and qualitative methods in a mixed methods study.
- **Priority or weighting:** The relative importance of the quantitative and qualitative methods for answering a mixed methods study's research questions.
- **Inferences:** The integrated study conclusions that are developed based on the interpretation of the quantitative and qualitative results in response to a research question.

THE ROLE OF THE MIXED METHODS RESEARCH PROCESS IN THE FIELD OF MIXED METHODS RESEARCH

As discussed in Chapter 1, when you read or review mixed methods studies, or design, conduct, and disseminate mixed methods research, you engage in a type of mixed methods research practice. Recall that mixed methods research practice includes any application of mixed methods research in advocating for, planning, conducting, disseminating, and evaluating the mixed methods research approach by researchers, scholars, and other stakeholders. At the core of all of these mixed methods research practices are the procedural issues related to the process of using mixed methods to address specific research purposes. For example, you need to consider these procedural issues when you read published mixed methods studies, plan and apply mixed methods to your own topic of interest, or review and evaluate mixed methods research done by others. In each of these situations, you will reflect on how the mixed methods research approach was used or can be used to address a posed research question and how its use is justified in the context of a particular study and its research topic.

In every application of mixed methods research, there are many factors that influence the decisions about the use of mixed methods, which result in different ways for how you form your knowledge about the mixed methods research process and how you approach mixed methods research practice. That is why we view the mixed methods research process as being at the core of our socio-ecological framework for mixed methods research, as introduced in Chapter 1. Just as your mixed methods research practice is focused on the use of mixed methods to address specific research purposes, the entire field of mixed methods research is also focused on the effective use of mixed methods to draw meaningful conclusions that address important research purposes. This central role of the mixed methods research process within mixed methods research practice and within the field is depicted in Figure 2.1. This process is

Figure 2.1   The Role of the Mixed Methods Research Process in the Practice of Mixed Methods Research

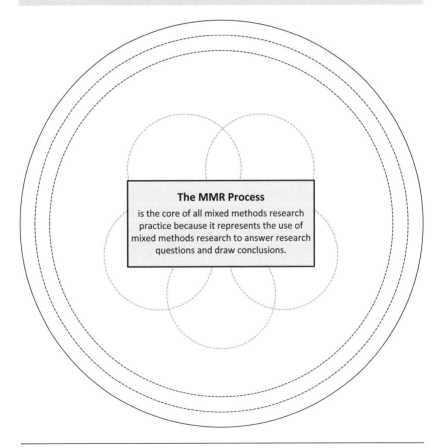

NOTE: MMR = mixed methods research.

anything but simple because it requires researchers to make different sets of decisions about how to use mixed methods to address research questions and draw conclusions. In addition, these decisions are informed and shaped by mixed methods research content considerations and a dynamic system of hierarchical personal, interpersonal, and social contexts. Before you can understand how these multiple factors interrelate with each other and jointly influence the way researchers apply mixed methods in their research practice, however, it is essential to first examine and gain an understanding of the process of mixed methods research, its basic components, and its associated practical issues.

MAJOR PERSPECTIVES ABOUT THE MIXED METHODS RESEARCH PROCESS

Research is a process of generating information in response to a research question, and the focus of the field of mixed methods research is ultimately about understanding the process of using mixed methods research to address research questions. We consider the **mixed methods research process** to be a process of research where researchers integrate quantitative and qualitative methods of data collection and analysis to best understand a research purpose (Creswell & Plano Clark, 2011). As we discussed in the previous section, the mixed methods research process is the how-to of mixed methods research practice because it underlies any process of advocating for, planning, conducting, disseminating, and evaluating a mixed methods research approach in an attempt to answer the posed research questions.

Most discussions about and applications of the mixed methods research process found in the literature are organized by the major steps involved in conducting research. Teddlie and Tashakkori (2009) differentiated three stages for considering the mixed methods research process: (1) conceptualization stage, during which the research purpose and questions that will guide the study are developed; (2) methods or experiential stage, during which the study is implemented and the data are collected and analyzed; and (3) inferential stage, during which the inferences from the quantitative and qualitative results or the integrated study conclusions are developed. We view these stages as integral components of the mixed methods research process and show their conceptual relationship in Figure 2.2. In practice, the relationship between the components of the research process can be more dynamic and interactive than indicated in the figure because researchers may also consider and adapt the study's research questions in response to the study's methods and generated

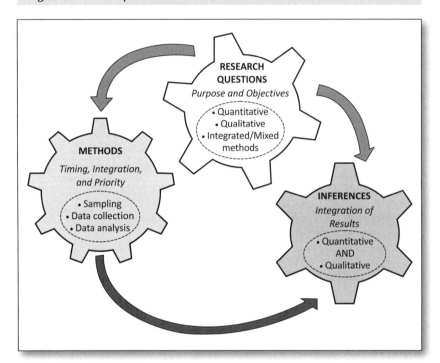

Figure 2.2   Components of the Mixed Methods Research Process

inferences (Maxwell & Loomis, 2003). We discuss each component and its role in the mixed methods research process in the following sections. In the later chapters, we emphasize the many considerations and contexts that influence the mixed methods research process, but here we discuss only its key components: research purpose and questions, methods, and inferences.

Research Purpose and Questions

Conceptualization of a mixed methods study begins with researchers specifying a research purpose (or research objectives) and formulating the research questions that they want to answer by implementing the study. The **research purpose and objectives** are statements of intent that identify the goals that researchers plan to achieve by undertaking a study. In some disciplines, such as the health sciences, funding agencies often require

researchers to state *specific aims,* which explicitly outline the key steps necessary to achieve a study objective. The research purpose and objectives play an
important role in a mixed methods study because they provide a foundation for
integrating the quantitative and qualitative methods to address one content aim
(Teddlie & Tashakkori, 2009). For example, Buck, Cook, Quigley, Eastwood,
and Lucas (2009) stated the following research purpose to guide their mixed
methods study of African American low-income girls' attitudes to learning
science discussed in Chapter 1 (see Box 1.1):

> The purpose of this initial study was to explore the attitudes toward
> science of urban African American girls from low SES communities
> using a mixed methods sequential explanatory design. (p. 391)

In the mixed methods study of factors influencing choices for colorectal
cancer screening also discussed in Chapter 1 (see Box 1.2), Ruffin, Creswell,
Jimbo, and Fetters (2009) provided the following objective that directed their
study procedures:

> The goal was to guide the development of a web-based tool to help
> patients choose among the screening options and then test the tool in
> a randomized controlled trial. (p. 80)

A study's research purpose and objectives are further refined into specific
research questions. **Research questions** help narrow researchers' ideas about
the content area of interest to specific questions that will be answered by collecting and analyzing the data in a study. In quantitative studies, researchers often
use *hypotheses statements,* which contain predictions about the outcomes of a
relationship among variables. Research questions are an important starting point
in the mixed methods research process because they set the boundaries to the
study, clarify its specific directions, and influence the selection of the research
methods (Plano Clark & Badiee, 2010; Teddlie & Tashakkori, 2009). A typical
mixed methods study has two sets of research questions: quantitative questions
and hypotheses that address the numeric aspect of the study and qualitative
questions that target the narrative information. Additionally, researchers may ask
an integrated question (Teddlie & Tashakkori, 2009)—also referred to as a mixed
methods research question (Creswell & Plano Clark, 2011; Onwuegbuzie &
Leech, 2006). The integrated research question addresses an overall intent of the

study and underscores the integration of the quantitative and qualitative methods in the process of the study implementation.

Box 2.1 presents the three types of research questions that Buck and colleagues (2009) used to guide their mixed methods study. These research questions directed the selection of the study participants, the methods of quantitative (survey) and qualitative (interview) data collection and analysis, and the integration of the quantitative and qualitative results.

Box 2.1

Research Questions in Buck et al.'s (2009) Mixed Methods Study of African American Girls' Attitudes to Learning Science

Quantitative Research Questions

1. Did the students in the sample score differently on the scales of the attitudes toward science survey?
2. What attitudes-toward-science profiles emerge from the scores on the attitudes toward science survey?

Qualitative Research Questions

1. What are the urban, low SES, African American girls' attitudes toward science and science learning?
2. What aspects of their experiences and understandings contribute to differences in attitudes?

Mixed Methods Question

1. How can the understandings that emerge from the qualitative data be used to provide a deeper understanding of the attitude-toward-science profiles?

Source: Adapted from Buck, G., Cook, K., Quigley, C., Eastwood, J., & Lucas, Y. (2009). Profiles of urban, low SES, African American girls' attitudes toward science: A sequential explanatory mixed methods study. *Journal of Mixed Methods Research, 3*(4), 386–410.

Methods

The research purpose and questions guide all methods decisions that researchers have to make during the experiential stage of a mixed methods study. These include decisions related to choosing the study design, selecting sampling strategies, identifying types of quantitative and qualitative data, and specifying methods of data analysis. In addition to these methods decisions that are common to any research process, including quantitative, qualitative, and mixed methods, there are other methods considerations that are specific to the mixed methods research process. Creswell and Plano Clark (2011) referred to these considerations as "key decisions" (p. 63) that researchers make when designing and implementing a mixed methods study. They include decisions about the timing or sequence of quantitative and qualitative data collection and analysis, integration or mixing of quantitative and qualitative data sets and subsequent results, and priority or weighting that each method carries in the study. These practical considerations of timing, integration, and priority have received extensive attention in the field of mixed methods research because they play an important role in guiding researchers' decisions about how to design and conduct a mixed methods study so that it produces meaningful inferences in response to the posed research questions.

Timing

In a mixed methods study, researchers can collect and analyze quantitative and qualitative data either at the same time or one following the other. **Timing or sequence** is the temporal relationship between the quantitative and qualitative components of data collection and analysis in a mixed methods study (Creswell & Plano Clark, 2011). Timing may be concurrent or sequential.

Concurrent timing implies that researchers collect and analyze both quantitative and qualitative data at the same time or independent from each other. For example, researchers can concurrently collect and analyze the data from a quantitative survey and qualitative individual interviews and then compare both sets of results. In Ruffin and colleagues' (2009) study, the researchers used concurrent timing when they independently collected and analyzed quantitative data from the survey with 93 participants and qualitative information from the focus groups with the same individuals. The decision to use concurrent timing was guided by the fact that the researchers wanted to have a more complete understanding of the factors influencing the choices of a colorectal cancer screening test by interpreting the focus group and survey results together.

Sequential timing refers to situations when researchers collect and analyze quantitative and qualitative data in sequence—one following or dependent on the other. For example, researchers can collect and analyze quantitative data first and then use these results to inform the follow-up qualitative data collection. Alternatively, researchers can first collect and analyze qualitative data to inform the subsequent quantitative data collection. In each case, researchers use the initial set of results to help determine what qualitative or quantitative data to collect next. Buck and colleagues (2009) used sequential timing in their study. They first collected and analyzed quantitative survey data to create four attitudes-toward-science profiles of 89 girls based on the scores that measured their attitudes toward science. Subsequently, they conducted qualitative interviews with 30 girls from grades 4 through 6, with 10 from each grade, to further explore and explain how four profiles reflecting students' personality orientations are related to their success in school and their experiences with science. The decision to use sequential timing was guided by the fact that the researchers wanted to first quantitatively identify different profiles of African American girls based on their attitudes to science and then to qualitatively explore how these profiles may explain the girls' engagement with science.

Integration

Integration is an essential component of the mixed methods research process (Teddlie & Tashakkori, 2006). The way researchers integrate quantitative and qualitative data and results in a study has implications for how researchers generate answers to the posed integrated research questions and develop inferences from the quantitative and qualitative results. **Integration or mixing** is an explicit interrelating of the quantitative and qualitative methods in a mixed methods study (Creswell & Plano Clark, 2011). Morse and Niehaus (2009) referred to the point in a study's implementation where the quantitative and qualitative methods join as "the point of interface" (p. 25). By using this term, they highlighted the importance of mixing quantitative and qualitative methods in producing integrated study conclusions.

The two most common integration approaches discussed in the literature include *combining* quantitative and qualitative sets of results during their joint interpretation at the completion of respective data collection and analysis and *connecting* quantitative and qualitative methods during data collection, when the results from the first quantitative or qualitative phase are used to inform the design and data collection of the subsequent qualitative or quantitative phase. For example, Ruffin and colleagues (2009), who used concurrent timing to collect and analyze quantitative and qualitative data, combined the results from the quantitative survey and qualitative focus group discussions to interpret them together. By integrating the different results in this combined way, the researchers were able to better understand factors that influence individuals' choices of colorectal screening test and to provide more complete answers to the study's research questions. Alternatively, Buck and colleagues (2009) connected the two sequential study phases when they used the attitudes-toward-science profiles created for 89 girls to inform the qualitative interviews with 30 purposefully selected girls to better understand and explain the reasons for the differences in the profiles. By integrating the quantitative and qualitative methods in this connected manner, the researchers were able to first identify the typical attitudes-toward-science profiles and then to explore each of these profiles in their relationship to girls' science achievement in more-depth.

Priority

Quantitative and qualitative methods can have different priority or carry different weight in a mixed methods study. **Priority** or **weighting** refers to the relative importance of the quantitative and qualitative methods for answering a mixed methods study's research questions (Creswell & Plano Clark, 2011). A mixed methods study can have either a *quantitative priority* when researchers place more emphasis on the quantitative data collection and analysis, a *qualitative priority* when researchers place more emphasis on the qualitative data collection and analysis, or *equal priority* when both types of data play an equally important role in answering a study's research questions. Researchers' knowledge and skills with quantitative and qualitative methods, access to participants and data, and available resources may also influence which method is prioritized in a mixed methods study.

For example, Buck and colleagues (2009) gave more priority to the quantitative data because they first had to create the attitudes-toward-science profiles of 89 girls and then "to use qualitative results to assist in explaining and interpreting quantitative findings" (p. 392). The researchers' decision was consistent with their mixed methods research question in that they wanted to gain better understanding of the four quantitative profiles, so the qualitative data performed a secondary role in the study. Whereas Ruffin and colleagues (2009) assigned more priority to the qualitative focus group data even though they collected and analyzed quantitative and qualitative data concurrently. Their decision was evidently guided by the fact that the qualitative data would yield more rich information about individuals' perceptions of colorectal cancer risk and screening preferences, which would better address their study's objective of informing a web-based tool to help patients choose among the screening options.

Inferences

The implementation of a mixed methods study culminates in the development of inferences, which we view as the goals and outcomes of the mixed methods research process. **Inferences** are integrated study conclusions that are developed based on the interpretation of the quantitative and qualitative results in response to a research question (Teddlie & Tashakkori, 2009). The process of generating inferences involves critically reviewing the results from the quantitative and qualitative data analyses in terms of how they jointly provide the answers to the study's research questions. This process is dynamic and is guided by the research questions, as reflected in Figure 2.2. It also involves researchers examining the relevance and quality of the collected data because they affect the overall quality of the study inferences that are produced from the integrated quantitative and qualitative results. We will discuss the issues of quality as they relate to the mixed methods research process in Chapter 7.

As an example of the process for developing inferences, Ruffin and colleagues (2009) generated inferences about individuals' choices of colorectal cancer screening test by combining survey results related to participants' knowledge and beliefs about colorectal cancer and focus group findings about participants' perceptions of colorectal cancer risk and screening preferences. Similarly, Buck and colleagues (2009) integrated the qualitative findings from their follow-up interviews with girls representing the four different attitudes-toward-science profiles with the quantitative descriptions of these profiles to develop inferences about the attitudes to learning science of African American girls from low socioeconomic status (SES) communities.

ISSUES AND DEBATES ABOUT THE MIXED METHODS RESEARCH PROCESS

Since the mixed methods research process reflects the core steps for conducting mixed methods research starting from research questions, to selection of methods and study implementation, and to study results and inferences, there is much consensus about what constitutes a process of conducting a mixed methods study. However, there are also some disagreements about the components of the mixed methods research process in the mixed methods literature. Here, we briefly introduce these issues that continue to be discussed and debated within the field of mixed methods research.

1. How should research questions be framed in a mixed methods study? Although most scholars view research questions as an integral component of the mixed methods research process, there are two opposing perspectives on writing research questions for a mixed methods study (Tashakkori & Creswell, 2007a; Teddlie & Tashakkori, 2009). The first perspective advocates for writing separate quantitative and qualitative research questions, which guide the implementation of the respective quantitative and qualitative study components, and a final mixed methods question that addresses the integration component of the entire study (Creswell & Plano Clark, 2007, 2011; Plano Clark & Badiee, 2010). This perspective supports the idea that a mixed methods question is necessary because it foreshadows the mixing of the quantitative and qualitative methods in the process of the study implementation. In contrast, the other perspective promotes using a single overarching integrated research question, which incorporates sub-questions for both quantitative and qualitative components of the study (Onwuegbuzie & Leech, 2006; Teddlie & Tashakkori, 2009; Yin, 2006). According to this perspective, an overarching research question helps justify the choice of the mixed methods design and helps align the study's research purpose, questions, and methods. You can find examples of authors having used both types of questions when you read mixed methods studies and can choose to include either or both of these perspectives when you write one or more mixed methods or integrated questions for your mixed methods study.

2. What is the real meaning of timing of quantitative and qualitative methods in the mixed methods research process? There is consensus in the mixed methods literature that the timing of quantitative and qualitative methods is an essential component of a mixed methods study implementation process. However, scholars use different terms and assign different meanings to the idea of timing. For example, Morse and Niehaus (2009) discussed *pacing* as "the synchronization of the core component and the supplementary component" in the context of the methods' integration

(p. 47). Decisions that researchers make about how to pace these components have implications for how quantitative and qualitative methods are integrated in a study. Other scholars view *timing* with reference to whether quantitative and qualitative methods are implemented concurrently or sequentially in a study (Greene, 2007; Teddlie & Tashakkori, 2009) or as a temporal relationship between the quantitative and qualitative study components (Creswell & Plano Clark, 2011). These scholars believe that decisions about timing are important considerations for the choice of a mixed methods study design. Some scholars prefer to think of *sequencing* of the two methods based on how the quantitative and qualitative results are used in a study to answer the research questions rather than the order in which the quantitative and qualitative data are collected in a study (Morgan, 2014). Whatever term you select to refer to timing in a mixed methods research study should be justified and supported by relevant literature so that the meaning is clear.

3. How should priority of the quantitative or qualitative methods be considered in the mixed methods research process? Priority is one of the most debatable issues related to the mixed methods research process. Different opinions exist about its practical importance and even whether considerations of priority should be included in the design and conduct of a mixed methods study. A related debatable point is whether the weight that different quantitative and qualitative methods carry in a study *can ever* be equal or whether they *should always* be of equal importance. In addition, scholars use different terms—for example, *weighting, emphasis, status, dominance* or *theoretical drive*—when they refer to the priority of the quantitative and qualitative methods in a study. Several scholars consider priority as an important dimension in the design and conduct of any mixed methods study (Creswell & Plano Clark, 2011; Morgan, 2014; Morse & Niehaus, 2009). Alternatively, Teddlie and Tashakkori (2009) argued that priority of the method cannot be completely determined before the study is implemented and thus should not be viewed as an important consideration of the mixed methods research process. Often priority can shift from one method to another based on the need to better understand the studied phenomenon and/or emergent study results. With these many different perspectives, you need to make an informed decision about whether to consider priority in guiding your thinking about designing and implementing a mixed methods study and make your viewpoint clear for your audiences.

4. What is the process of drawing quality inferences in a mixed methods study? Tashakkori and Teddlie (2003a, 2010b) referred to drawing quality inferences in mixed methods studies as one of the major controversies of mixed methods research. Although inferences are the most important aspect of a mixed methods study, an important issue is that the process of making inferences and description of their essential features have received little attention in the mixed methods literature. Due to its origin in philosophy, the term *inferences* has different meanings outside of the field of research methodology. Sometimes researchers do not clearly differentiate between the study results and inferences, or inferences are not seen as distinct integrated study conclusions (Tashakkori & Teddlie, 2010b). Additionally, some researchers from a qualitative research orientation believe that the term *inferences* has a strong quantitative connotation since it is associated with statistical analysis (Creswell, 2010). You should carefully consider all these views when approaching the process of drawing inferences in your mixed methods research practice.

These four questions highlight important issues and debates related to the major components of the mixed methods research process. They also indicate the importance for researchers to clearly define their position in how they view the process of mixed methods research, what research questions they choose to guide it, and what they consider to be the outcomes of mixing quantitative and qualitative methods in the process of a study's implementation. These and other debates about the mixed methods research process contribute to the complexity of mixed methods research but at the same time open up opportunities for flexibility and creativity. As Teddlie and Tashakkori (2009) observed, "Making inferences is both an art and a science" (p. 289).

APPLYING THE MIXED METHODS RESEARCH PROCESS IN RESEARCH PRACTICE

At its essence, the entire field of mixed methods research is about the mixed methods research process that researchers use to address certain types of research questions and to develop inferences grounded in the integrated study results. At the heart of this process are the basic components that describe the research purpose, questions, methods, and inferences involved when quantitative and qualitative methods are integrated in a mixed methods study. Recognizing and describing these components is essential for understanding the planning, conducting, reporting, and evaluating of mixed methods studies. Box 2.2 includes our advice for applying the concepts of this chapter to your mixed methods research practice.

Box 2.2

Advice for Applying the Mixed Methods Research Process in Research Practice

Advice for Reading/Reviewing Mixed Methods Studies and Methodological Discussions

- Identify the authors' overall intent and research questions, paying attention to which methods (quantitative, qualitative, or both) are needed to address each question.
- Note whether the authors explicitly stated the research purpose and questions, including the research questions for the quantitative and qualitative study components and an integrated or mixed methods research question.
- Note whether the authors explained if any of the research questions emerged during the implementation of the study.
- Assess how the authors addressed the issues of timing (concurrent or sequential), integration (combined or connected), and priority (equal or unequal) of the quantitative and qualitative methods in the study and whether the authors explained what guided their decisions.
- Assess how the issues of timing, integration, and priority guided the authors' approaches to sampling, data collection, and data analysis in the study.
- Assess how the authors addressed the integration of the quantitative and qualitative methods in the context of the study's research questions.
- Note whether the reported inferences or integrated conclusions were guided by the study's research questions and provide answers to those questions.

Advice for Proposing/Reporting/Discussing Mixed Methods Research

- Explicitly state your research purpose and specific research questions, including the research questions for the quantitative and qualitative study components and an integrated or mixed methods research question.
- Make it clear to the reader which research questions call for the use of which methods (quantitative, qualitative, or both).
- Note if any of the research questions emerged during the implementation of the study, and if so, explain how they emerged.
- Provide a clear definition of timing, integration, and priority of the quantitative and qualitative methods, and explain how you addressed these issues and what influenced your decisions.
- Explain how the issues of timing, integration, and priority guided your approaches to sampling, data collection, and data analysis in the study.
- Explain what role the integration of the quantitative and qualitative methods played in the context of the posed research questions in your study.
- Discuss the process of developing the inferences or integrated conclusions and how it was guided by the study's research questions.

When reading and reviewing the literature about mixed methods research, it is essential to pay particular attention to how the authors used the mixed methods research process and how they addressed its basic components. As you read and evaluate the mixed methods literature, try to identify the authors' overall intent for using mixed methods. Also note how the authors stated the research purpose, or objectives, and the research questions for the quantitative, qualitative, and integrated study components. When research questions are stated explicitly and clearly, they can help you better understand what guided the authors' decisions in choosing the study's methods related to sampling, data collection, and data analysis. It is also important to understand how the authors addressed the issues of timing, integration, and priority of the quantitative and qualitative methods in the study in the context of the posed research questions and how the generated inferences help answer these questions.

It is particularly important to appropriately address the components of the mixed methods research process when designing and reporting your own mixed methods research study. Readers who will review and evaluate your study will benefit from a clear statement of the research purpose or objectives, research questions, and a detailed discussion about the study's methods. It is also important to be clear about how you frame your integrated or mixed methods research question—as a single overarching research question that incorporates sub-questions for both quantitative and qualitative components or as an integrated question that addresses mixing of the quantitative and qualitative methods in the process of the study implementation. It is equally important to explain if any of the research questions emerged during the conduct of the study and if you had to make any adjustments in the study's methods in response to these questions. Readers who are new to mixed methods research will also benefit if you provide a clear definition of timing, integration, and priority and explain how you address these issues and what influenced your decisions. You also need to be explicit in how you develop inferences as your mixed methods study outcomes and how they provide answers to the posed research questions. By fully explaining the basic components of the mixed methods research process, your readers will be in a better position to understand and evaluate your mixed methods research practice.

CONCLUDING COMMENTS

We conclude the chapter by offering some final summary comments organized by the learning objectives stated at the beginning of the chapter.

- **Describe the components in the mixed methods research process that is the core of mixed methods research practice.** The mixed methods research process is the centerpiece of the socio-ecological framework for mixed methods research and encompasses the procedural issues related to the use of mixed methods to address specific research purposes and draw meaningful conclusions. The mixed methods research process is the core and how-to of mixed methods research practice and consists of three stages: conceptualization, experiential or methods, and inferential. This process is of central importance when reading about, conducting, evaluating, teaching, and advocating for mixed methods research.

- **Understand the role of the research purpose, objectives, and questions in the mixed methods research process.** The research purpose and objectives identify the goals researchers plan to achieve by undertaking a study. In a mixed methods study, the research purpose and questions also provide a foundation for integrating quantitative and qualitative methods to address one content aim. A typical mixed methods study includes quantitative research questions that address the numeric aspect of the study and qualitative research questions that target the narrative information. An integrated or mixed methods question addresses an overall intent of the study and emphasizes the integration of the quantitative and qualitative methods in the process of the study implementation.

- **Consider the practical issues related to the use of methods in the mixed methods research process, such as timing, integration, and priority.** The practical considerations of timing, integration, and priority play an important role in guiding researchers' decisions about how to design and conduct a mixed methods study so that it produces meaningful inferences in response to the posed research questions. These decisions relate to whether to collect and analyze quantitative and qualitative data concurrently or sequentially; how to integrate quantitative and qualitative data in the process of the study implementation by means of combining or connecting; and what method, quantitative or qualitative, or both to give priority in the study.

- **Explain the nature of inferences that are the outcome of the mixed methods research process.** The development of inferences or integrated study conclusions are the goals and outcomes of the mixed methods research process. Researchers develop inferences by interpreting the results from the quantitative and qualitative data analyses with regard to how they jointly provide the answers to the posed research questions.

APPLICATION QUESTIONS

1. Reflect on the role of the mixed methods research process in the practice of mixed methods research. Why do you think the mixed methods research process forms the core of mixed methods research practice and why it is viewed as the centerpiece of the socio-ecological framework for mixed methods research?

2. Locate a published mixed methods study in your discipline or area of interest. Carefully read the study reflecting on how the study was conceptualized, designed, and conducted. Discuss the components of the mixed methods research process described in the study:

   a. The research purpose, objectives, and questions that guided the study. If the authors stated the research questions, identify the type of questions as quantitative, qualitative, and mixed methods.

   b. The authors' approach to the issues of timing, integration, and priority of the quantitative and qualitative methods in the study.

   c. The inferences that emerged from the study in response to the research questions and how well they are grounded in the quantitative and qualitative results.

3. Choose one question from the ongoing issues and debates about the mixed methods research process discussed in this chapter. State why you selected that question, and discuss your reactions to it in terms of its relationship to the mixed methods research process. Do you think this issue warrants further discussion and debate? Justify your answer.

4. Carefully read our advice for applying the mixed methods research process in mixed methods research practice in Box 2.1. Identify the role that would best describe how you apply mixed methods in your research practice (e.g., as a reader, reviewer, researcher, evaluator, or instructor), and discuss how you will use our advice to guide your mixed methods research practice.

KEY RESOURCES

To learn more about the components of the mixed methods research process, we suggest you start with the following resources:

*1. Tashakkori, A., & Creswell, J. W. (2007). Exploring the nature of research questions in mixed methods research [Editorial]. *Journal of Mixed Methods Research, 1*(3), 207–211.

- In this editorial, Tashakkori and Creswell addressed the nature of mixed research questions. The editors discussed different perspectives about research questions in mixed methods research and provided suggestions for the type of questions researchers should consider including in mixed methods studies.

2. **Creswell, J. W., & Plano Clark, V. L. (2011). Key decisions in choosing a mixed methods design. In** *Designing and conducting mixed methods research* **(2nd ed., pp. 63–68). Thousand Oaks, CA: Sage.**

   - In this part of the chapter from Creswell and Plano Clark's book, the authors described four methodological considerations that are inherent to the mixed methods research process: priority, timing, and integration of the quantitative and qualitative methods as well as the level of interaction between the quantitative and qualitative components.

*3. **Bazeley, P., & Kemp, L. (2012). Mosaics, triangles, and DNA: Metaphors for integrated analysis in mixed methods research.** *Journal of Mixed Methods Research, 6*(1), 55–72.

   - In this article, Bazeley and Kemp analyzed the different ways researchers describe the integrative processes used in mixed methods studies and suggested eight principles and strategies for effective methods' integration in mixed methods research.

4. **Teddlie, C., & Tashakkori, A. (2009). The inference process in mixed methods research. In** *Foundations of mixed methods research: Integrating quantitative and qualitative approaches in the social and behavioral sciences* **(pp. 285–314). Thousand Oaks, CA: Sage.**

   - In this chapter from Teddlie and Tashakkori's book, the authors discussed the nature of inferences in mixed methods research and the process by which researchers make quality inferences when integrating quantitative and qualitative study results.

---

* The key resource is available at the following website: http://study.sagepub.com/planoclark.

PART II

METHODOLOGICAL CONTENT CONSIDERATIONS FOR MIXED METHODS RESEARCH PRACTICE

We now turn our focus to the methodological content considerations that directly influence how scholars use mixed methods in their research practice. Recall that the mixed methods content considerations form the middle layer of our socio-ecological framework for the field of mixed methods research. These mixed methods content domains are shaped by personal, interpersonal, and social contexts and come together to directly influence the mixed methods research process. They represent the prominent content considerations discussed in the field, which aim to answer five basic questions about mixed methods research: (1) What is it? (2) Why use it? (3) How to use it? (4) How to combine it with other approaches? (5) How to assess it? In the chapters that follow in Part II, we examine each of these content domains by presenting the major perspectives that exist, highlighting important issues and debates among those perspectives, providing examples of how the perspectives are demonstrated in mixed methods research practice, and offering recommendations for applying the content domain to your mixed methods research practice. The five chapters in Part II are as follows:

Chapter 3: What Is Mixed Methods Research? Considering How Mixed
  Methods Research Is Defined
Chapter 4: Why Use Mixed Methods Research? Identifying Rationales for
  Mixing Methods
Chapter 5: How to Use Mixed Methods Research? Understanding the Basic
  Mixed Methods Designs

Chapter 6: How to Expand the Use of Mixed Methods Research?
        Intersecting Mixed Methods With Other Approaches
Chapter 7: How to Assess Mixed Methods Research? Considering Mixed
        Methods Research Quality

THREE

WHAT IS MIXED METHODS RESEARCH?

CONSIDERING HOW MIXED METHODS RESEARCH IS DEFINED

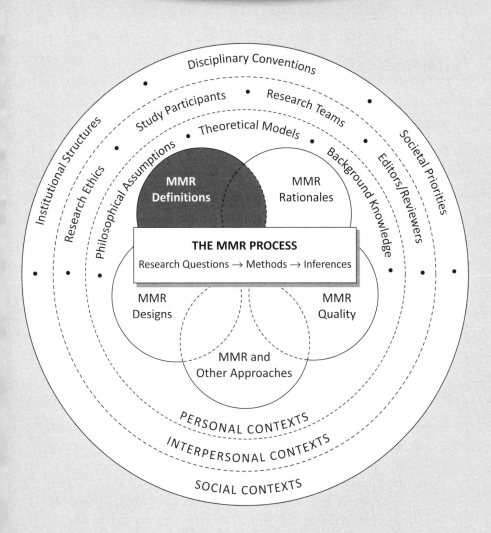

When you first heard the words mixed methods research, *you probably asked, What is it? Similarly, the field of mixed methods research has been grappling with how to define mixed methods from its beginning as well. Today the field encompasses a rich (and often bewildering) landscape of terminology and perspectives that have resulted in a variety of ways to define and think about mixed methods research. Although these many definitions can be perplexing at times for those new to mixed methods research, in the end they serve to enhance the breadth and inclusiveness of the field in important ways. Therefore, it is helpful to consider the nuances of how mixed methods is defined so that you can effectively understand the different perspectives present in the field.*

LEARNING OBJECTIVES

This chapter aims to provide you with an understanding of how mixed methods research is defined so you are able to do the following:

- Understand commonly used terminology for defining mixed methods research.
- Identify the different ways that mixed methods research is defined, and consider the implications of these differences for mixed methods research practice.
- Articulate the definition for mixed methods research that aligns with your perspectives about mixing methods.

CHAPTER 3 KEY CONCEPTS

The following key concepts will help you navigate through the main considerations related to defining mixed methods research as they are introduced in this chapter:

- **Mixed methods research:** A term used for the process of research when researchers integrate quantitative methods of data collection and analysis and qualitative methods of data collection and analysis.
- **Mixed research:** A term used for the process of research when researchers integrate at least one quantitative approach and at least one qualitative approach.

- **Multimethod research:** A term used for the process of research when researchers integrate multiple quantitative approaches, multiple qualitative approaches, or multiple quantitative and qualitative approaches.
- **Methods:** Procedures or techniques used to implement the sampling, data collection, or data analysis steps within a research study.
- **Methodology:** The process of research from formulating questions to drawing conclusions in a study.
- **Philosophy (or paradigm or mental model):** The collection of assumptions and values about the nature of reality and knowledge that provide the foundation for a research study.
- **Communities of research practice:** Groups of scholars who share common beliefs, agendas, and substantive knowledge related to the conduct of research.

THE ROLE OF DEFINITIONS IN THE FIELD OF MIXED METHODS RESEARCH

As introduced in Chapter 1, mixed methods research is at its essence the intentional integration of quantitative and qualitative research approaches to best address a research problem. A definition such as this serves many purposes. Mixed methods research needs to be definable, with a recognized name and meaning associated with that name, to be considered a distinctive and legitimate approach to research (Greene, 2008; Johnson, Onwuegbuzie, & Turner, 2007; Teddlie & Tashakkori, 2003). Such a definition distinguishes mixed methods research from other approaches and facilitates communication about its use. When researchers are able to invoke a recognizable name and definition for their research approach, it often enhances the acceptability of that approach within their research communities. Therefore, being able to define mixed methods is essential for any types of mixed methods research practice you engage in as a reader, reviewer, researcher, or instructor of mixed methods.

The importance of defining mixed methods research goes beyond using particular terminology, however. As suggested by the conceptual framework for mixed methods research we advanced in Chapter 1, the definition of mixed methods research is an important methodological content consideration for mixed methods research practice. Scholars use a variety of terms to define mixed methods research, and they bring different ideas about what "counts" as *quantitative, qualitative,* and *integration,* which are the essential elements of mixed methods. These differences reflect the influence of different personal, interpersonal, and social contexts that shape scholars' use of mixed methods research. We will discuss the details of these definitional differences later in this chapter, but first it is useful to consider the implication of such differences. Figure 3.1 emphasizes how the definition of mixed methods research directly shapes the mixed methods research process. This means that differences in definitions can manifest as differences in the ways that researchers apply mixed methods research when they state their research questions, choose their methods, and draw inferences. Therefore, you need to be able to recognize and

Figure 3.1   The Role of Definitions in the Practice of Mixed Methods Research

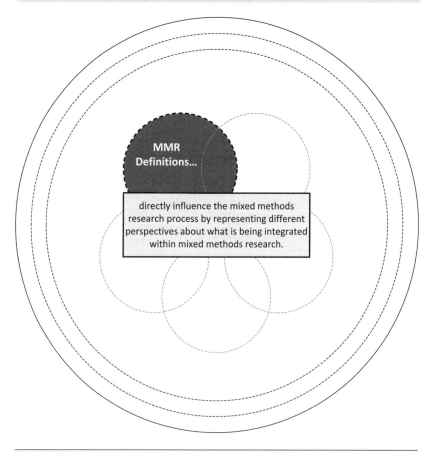

MMR Definitions...

directly influence the mixed methods research process by representing different perspectives about what is being integrated within mixed methods research.

NOTE: MMR = mixed methods research.

distinguish different mixed methods definitions because they have important implications for understanding and using mixed methods research.

TERMINOLOGY USED
TO NAME MIXED METHODS RESEARCH

Mixed methods scholars have spent considerable attention and effort on choosing a name for this approach. Examples of terms that have been used include *mixed methods research* (no hyphen), *mixed-methods research* (with hyphen), *mixed method research* (no s), *mixed methodology, methodological triangulation, multimethod research, integrated research, combined research,* and *mixed research.* In their own way, each of these terms conveys the notion that two different approaches (i.e., quantitative and qualitative) are being brought together (i.e., integrated or mixed).

Although you can find scholars who continue to use each of the terms just listed (and more) today, the field has largely settled on the term *mixed methods research,* and this is the term that we have selected to use throughout this book. The prominence of this term was solidified with the publication of the first *Handbook of Mixed Methods in Social & Behavioral Research* in 2003 (Tashakkori & Teddlie, 2003a) and the debut of the *Journal of Mixed Methods Research* (JMMR) in 2007 (Tashakkori & Creswell, 2007b). The term **mixed methods research** has come to indicate a process of research when researchers integrate quantitative methods of data collection and analysis and qualitative methods of data collection and analysis to understand a research problem. Therefore, this term resonates with many scholars because it focuses on the combination of both quantitative and qualitative methods—the specific procedures and techniques used in a study. As such, this term provides a very concrete and practical way for identifying the field and the approach used in a particular study.

There are other names that have received considerable attention in the field of mixed methods research. For example, the term **mixed research** has gained support as a term used to indicate a process of research when researchers integrate at least one quantitative approach and at least one qualitative approach (Johnson & Onwuegbuzie, 2004). Many scholars prefer this term because they view it as more inclusive of a broader range of mixing possibilities (e.g., mixing different types of questions or mixing different forms of language) than requiring the mixing of both quantitative and qualitative data collection and analysis methods. Early on, the term **multimethod research** also gained some popularity to indicate the combination of two or more methods, particularly in the health sciences. However, many scholars of mixed methods research do not prefer this term because it emphasizes the use of different methods but not the integration (or mixing) aspect. Instead, we find that this term is currently being used to denote any combination of multiple methods within a study, including those from a single methodological approach (Hesse-Biber, 2010b; Morse & Niehaus, 2009). That is, the term *multimethod research* designates studies in which the researcher combines multiple quantitative approaches (e.g., experimental and survey research methods) or combines multiple qualitative approaches (e.g., ethnographic and narrative research methods) or combines both quantitative and qualitative approaches.

When reading or writing about mixed methods research, it is useful for you to note that the field has largely adopted the use of these three terms (*mixed methods research, mixed research,* and *multimethod research*), but other terminology continues to be used as well. In addition, you will find situations where scholars use the different terms interchangeably and other times where they use them to indicate important differences in the definitions of these terms as we have noted. Now, we turn our attention to further consider the different perspectives that exist for defining mixed methods research.

MAJOR PERSPECTIVES FOR DEFINING MIXED METHODS RESEARCH

As the brief introduction to terminology in the previous section foreshadowed, scholars bring a variety of perspectives to mixed methods research that shape how they define it. These perspectives include thinking of mixed methods research as a method, as a methodology, as a philosophy, and/or as a community of research practice. Drawing from Creswell (2010), we find it helpful to conceptualize these different perspectives that shape the many existing definitions of mixed methods research as shown in Figure 3.2. This figure emphasizes the four different dimensions or levels for thinking about what is being mixed within mixed methods research. In the paragraphs that follow, we discuss what it means to view mixed methods research from the perspectives of mixing methods, methodologies, philosophies, or communities of research practice.

A common way to define mixed methods research is based on the mixing of quantitative and qualitative methods. **Methods** are the specific procedures or techniques that are used to implement a research study. Examples of such methods

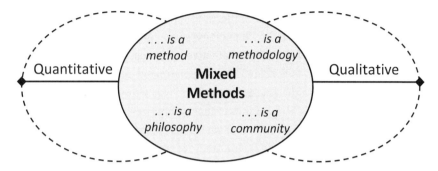

Figure 3.2   Different Perspectives for Defining Mixed Methods Research

are the procedures used for collecting data (e.g., repeated measures achievement test or nonparticipant observation) and analyzing data (e.g., statistical multilevel modeling or coding and thematic development). When scholars define mixed methods research in terms of methods, they focus on research approaches that combine methods of data collection and data analysis associated with quantitative research and methods of data collection and data analysis associated with qualitative research (e.g., Creswell & Plano Clark, 2007; Greene, Caracelli, & Graham, 1989). Defining mixed methods research in terms of methods is particularly practical when examining published research because researchers generally report their method procedures as part of their empirical study reports. For this reason, methods-based definitions are common in systematic reviews of the use of mixed methods (e.g., Bryman, 2006a; Plano Clark et al., 2014).

Another perspective for defining mixed methods research emphasizes the mixing of quantitative and qualitative approaches at the level of methodology. Here, we use the term ***methodology*** to indicate the full process of research from formulating questions to drawing conclusions in a study. That is, methodology includes the methods of a study but also includes the conceptualization and interpretation stages of the research process. Scholars who define mixed methods from this perspective often discuss mixing as occurring at one or more stages of the research process, such as mixing intents associated with both quantitative and qualitative approaches within a study's research questions (e.g., Johnson & Onwuegbuzie, 2004; Tashakkori & Teddlie, 1998). Whereas definitions that emphasize *methods* typically require studies to include both quantitative methods (i.e., data collection and data analysis) and qualitative methods (i.e., data collection and data analysis), definitions that emphasize a *methodology* perspective consider mixed methods to include studies that mix within and/or across the stages of the research process (i.e., research questions, design, data collection, data analysis, and/or interpretation). For example, a mixed methodology study might ask a quantitatively oriented research question, gather qualitative open-ended interview data, and then analyze the open-ended data using predetermined categories and statistical analyses to address the research question. Such a study would be considered as mixed methods by a definition that emphasizes mixing methodology because it mixed quantitative research questions and analyses with qualitative data collection. In contrast, this same study would not satisfy a definition of mixed methods that requires the mixing of quantitative data collection and analysis methods along with qualitative data collection and analysis methods.

Other scholars define mixed methods from a perspective that emphasizes philosophy. We use the term ***philosophy*** to mean a collection of assumptions and values about the nature of reality and knowledge that provide the foundation for a research study. Philosophy includes formal systems of beliefs (or paradigms) such as postpositivism, constructivism, and pragmatism, as well as more informal notions of mental models and conceptual frameworks that describe how researchers think about their topic and research. (Note, we will further consider philosophies as important personal contexts for mixed methods research in Chapter 8.) When scholars define mixed methods research from a philosophical perspective, they focus more on the idea of bringing different sets of beliefs and assumptions into dialogue with each other than on the idea of mixing particular techniques or in particular stages of research (e.g., Greene, 2007). Writings about mixed methods framed from the philosophical perspective have a different flavor to them than writings framed with a focus on the methods that researchers choose to use because the focus is as much or more on the philosophical assumptions informing the research as the method procedures used to do the research.

One final perspective used to define mixed methods research occurs when scholars consider communities of research practice. **Communities of research practice** are formal and informal groups of scholars who share common beliefs, research agendas, and substantive knowledge related to the conduct of research. When mixed methods research is defined from the perspective of research communities, it focuses on bringing together scholars who value and use quantitative and qualitative approaches in combination (e.g., Denscombe, 2008; Teddlie & Tashakkori, 2009). Members of this community may include groups of individuals who self-identify as mixed methods researchers or a team of researchers who individually self-identify as quantitative researchers or qualitative researchers and decide to work together on a mixed methods research project.

This discussion has emphasized that there are significant differences among the perspectives for defining mixed methods research in terms of methods, methodology, philosophy, or research communities. It is important to note that there is also a great deal of overlap in the notion of bringing together quantitative and qualitative approaches for research. Some examples of mixed methods research incorporate all of these perspectives by viewing mixing in terms of methods, methodology, philosophy, and communities of research practice. In those cases, it can be useful to consider and recognize the many different levels of mixing that are occurring. In other cases, however, the differences among these perspectives can result in debates and disagreements about what is and is not mixed methods research. These differences can lead to confusion, such as when some scholars label a certain approach as an example of what mixed methods research is and other scholars label the same approach as an example of what mixed methods research is not. These inconsistencies within the field can be perplexing unless you understand that they reflect different perspectives for defining mixed methods research.

EXAMPLES OF MIXED METHODS RESEARCH DEFINITIONS

To fully appreciate the different perspectives that exist for defining mixed methods research, it is helpful to consider examples for how these different perspectives manifest when scholars write about mixed methods research within the methodological literature and researchers report on their empirical research practice. Most formal definitions for mixed methods research emerge from the methodological literature in the field, and researchers generally draw from these available definitions to inform their own work. We provide examples of both types of mixed methods definitions in the sections that follow.

Definitions From the Methodological Literature

A wide array of definitions for mixed methods research is found in the methodological literature about mixed methods research. Table 3.1 introduces 10 of these definitions and offers our comments about the major perspectives

Table 3.1 Ten Definitions for Mixed Methods Research From the Methodological Literature

Authors [a]	Definition of Mixed Methods Research	Comments
Greene, Caracelli, and Graham (1989)	"We defined mixed-method designs as those that include at least one quantitative method (designed to collect numbers) and one qualitative method (designed to collect words), where neither type of method is inherently linked to any particular inquiry paradigm." (p. 256)	This definition: • emphasizes a *method* perspective. • is one of the earliest definitions found in the field. • is provided by authors trained in evaluation.
Johnson and Onwuegbuzie (2004)	"Mixed methods research is formally defined here as the class of research where the researcher mixes or combines quantitative and qualitative research techniques, methods, approaches, concepts or language into a single study." (p. 17)	This definition: • emphasizes a *methodology* perspective. • is provided by authors trained in education.
Creswell and Plano Clark (2007)	"*Mixed methods research* is a research design with philosophical assumptions as well as methods of inquiry. As a methodology, it involves philosophical assumptions that guide the direction of the collection and analysis of data and the mixture of qualitative and quantitative approaches in many phases in the research process. As a method, it focuses on collecting, analyzing, and mixing both quantitative and qualitative data in a single study or series of studies. Its central premise is that the use of quantitative and qualitative approaches in combination provides a better understanding of research problems than either approach alone." (p. 5)	This definition: • includes a *method* and *methodology* perspective. • is provided by authors trained in education.

| Greene (2007) | "The core meaning of mixing methods in social inquiry is to invite multiple mental models into the same inquiry space for purposes of respectful conversation, dialogue, and learning one from the other, toward a collective generation of better understanding of the phenomena being studied. By definition, then, mixed methods social inquiry involves a plurality of philosophical paradigms, theoretical assumptions, methodological traditions, data gathering and analysis techniques, and personalized understandings and value commitments—because these are the stuff of mental models." (p. 13) | This definition:
• emphasizes a *philosophy* perspective.
• is provided by an author trained in evaluation. |
| Tashakkori and Creswell (2007b) | "As an effort to be as inclusive as possible, we have broadly defined mixed methods here as research in which the investigator collects and analyzes data, integrates the findings, and draws inferences using both qualitative and quantitative approaches or methods in a single study or a program of inquiry." (p. 4) | This definition:
• emphasizes a *methodology* perspective.
• is provided by the founding editors for the *Journal of Mixed Methods Research* (JMMR), the leading journal in the field. |

(Continued)

Table 3.1 (Continued)

Authors [a]	Definition of Mixed Methods Research	Comments
Johnson, Onwuegbuzie, and Turner (2007)	"Mixed methods research is the type of research in which a researcher or team of researchers combines elements of qualitative and quantitative research approaches (e.g., use of qualitative and quantitative viewpoints, data collection, analysis, inference techniques) for the broad purposes of breadth and depth of understanding and corroboration." (p. 123)	This definition: • includes a *methodology* and *philosophy* perspective. • emerged from a study of 21 noted mixed methods scholars representing several disciplines.
Teddlie and Tashakkori (2009)	"We refer to [mixed methods research] as the *third research community* in this chapter because we are focusing on the relationships that exist within and among the three major groups that are currently doing research in the social and behavioral sciences. Mixed methods (MM) research has emerged as an alternative to the dichotomy of qualitative (QUAL) and quantitative (QUAN) traditions during the past 20 years." (p. 4)	This definition: • emphasizes a *community of research practice* perspective. • is provided by authors trained in social psychology.
Morse and Niehaus (2009)	"Mixed method research is therefore a systematic way of using two or more research methods to answer a single research question." (p. 9)	This definition: • emphasizes a *method* perspective. • is provided by authors trained in nursing.

66

Creswell, Klassen, Plano Clark, and Smith for the Office of Behavioral and Social Sciences Research (2011)	"For purposes of this discussion, mixed methods research will be defined as a research approach or methodology: • focusing on research questions that call for real-life contextual understandings, multi-level perspectives, and cultural influences; • employing rigorous quantitative research assessing magnitude and frequency of constructs and rigorous qualitative research exploring the meaning and understanding of constructs; • utilizing multiple methods (e.g., intervention trials and in-depth interviews); • intentionally integrating or combining these methods to draw on the strengths of each; and • framing the investigation within philosophical and theoretical positions." (p. 4)	This definition: • emphasizes a *methodology* perspective. • was developed for the field of health sciences by 18 members of a working group commissioned by the National Institutes of Health (NIH).
Morgan (2014)	Mixed methods research designs are "projects that collect both qualitative and quantitative data so that using the combined strengths of qualitative and quantitative methods will accomplish more than would have been possible with one method alone." (p. xiii)	This definition: • emphasizes a *method* perspective. • was developed by an author trained in sociology.

[a]Examples are listed in chronological order.

and contexts associated with each. We purposefully selected definitions found within the field that represent different perspectives for defining mixed methods research as a method, methodology, philosophy, and/or community. As our comments highlight, these definitions have emerged from scholars representing several different disciplines, including evaluation, education, sociology, and health sciences. The selected definitions are listed in chronological order and therefore also provide an idea of how the definitions of mixed methods research have evolved over time from the beginning of the field in the late 1980s to the time we are writing this book. In addition, the definitions listed in Table 3.1 include the most highly cited definitions found in the literature. Therefore, this collection provides a good overview of the available possibilities from which you can choose to define mixed methods research in your own research practice.

Definitions Used in Mixed Methods Research Studies

Researchers who mix methods in their empirical research studies also define this approach for their audiences—particularly if these audiences are unfamiliar with mixed methods research. Mirroring the variety represented in Table 3.1, researchers are drawn to different perspectives for defining a mixed methods approach in their research studies and use different rhetorical strategies for stating their definitions. One common approach is for researchers to offer a simple definition when first introducing the term into a study report. For example, Blakely, Skirton, Cooper, Allum, and Nelmes (2010) used this strategy in the report of their mixed methods study of educators' use of educational games. They wrote the following:

> We decided to conduct a "mixed-methods" study, comprising both qualitative and quantitative components. (p. 28)

Some definitions provided in empirical research articles focus on a particular stage of a study such as data collection or data analysis instead of the full research process. The definition stated by Mitchell (2010) for her mixed methods study of parental happiness is an example of this strategy. Her definition focused on mixing methods within the analysis stage of the research by stating the following:

> This data analysis combines a mixed methods approach by integrating statistical and thematic data analytic techniques. (p. 330)

Although many briefly stated definitions tend to emphasize the method or methodology perspective, there are also examples from researchers who bring a philosophical perspective to their definition. For example, Farquhar, Ewing, and Booth (2011) provided the following philosophy-based definition of mixed methods research for the report of their research to develop and evaluate interventions in palliative care:

> Mixed method research brings together quantitative and qualitative research methods from the different research paradigms of positivism and interpretivism. (p. 749)

Many researchers choose to use a more formal rhetorical style for defining mixed methods research by drawing on and citing specific definitions found in the methodological literature. For example, Lee and Greene (2007) combined multiple perspectives from the literature when they stated their definition of mixed methods research in a study about graduate students' performance as it relates to scores on an English as a second language placement test. They wrote the following:

> A mixed methods approach is considered by many to be a third methodological movement in educational and social research (Johnson et al., 2007), which rejects the "either-or" need to choose between quantitative and qualitative approaches (Tashakkori & Teddlie, 2003) and in fact explicitly calls for the integrated use of methods from diverse inquiry traditions. (p. 368)

When drawing from the methodological literature, some researchers base their definition of mixed methods research on writings from their specific discipline. For example, in the health sciences, some researchers have defined mixed methods research using the definition provided within a document commissioned by the National Institutes of Health (NIH; see Creswell et al., 2011, in Table 3.1). Peterson et al. (2013) used this strategy in their mixed methods study designed to test an intervention based in positive affect and self-affirmation. They stated the following:

> Mixed methods research comprises a participant-centered, culturally grounded set of techniques that employ, in tandem, methodologically rigorous quantitative and qualitative approaches in an integrated,

theory driven manner (Creswell, Klassen, Plano Clark, & Clegg Smith, 2011). (p. 218)

Whether demonstrating a more informal or formal rhetorical style, these examples illustrate different ways that researchers define mixed methods research and include their definitions in their study reports. These examples provide you with models for how you might incorporate the definition of mixed methods research into your mixed methods research practice.

ISSUES AND DEBATES ABOUT DEFINITIONS

Considering the many different perspectives that exist about mixed methods research, it should come as no surprise that there remain ongoing issues and debates about the definition of this research approach and the field that has emerged around it. Here, we briefly introduce four related issues that continue to be discussed and debated within the field.

1. What is *the* best definition for mixed methods research? As this chapter has demonstrated, there is *not* one accepted or best definition for mixed methods research despite the formal development of the field since the late 1980s (Denscombe, 2008; Johnson et al., 2007; Teddlie & Tashakkori, 2003). Although those new to the field often expect a high level of consensus for something as fundamental as the definition of mixed methods, many definitions continue to be used that reflect different perspectives about integrating at the level of methods, methodology, philosophy, and/or communities of research practice. The many definitions in use reflect the different personal perspectives and disciplinary contexts that scholars bring to the field, which we will discuss further in Chapters 8 through 10. Despite the lack of consensus, the available definitions provide you with a variety of options from which you can choose to use in your research practice.

2. Should there be *one* definition for mixed methods research? Scholars differ in their opinions about the value of having a single definition for mixed methods research. There are some who advocate for the members of the field reaching consensus regarding basic terminology and definitions for mixed methods research (Teddlie & Tashakkori, 2010). These scholars note that such agreement will facilitate communication and clarity. There are others, however, who advocate for the value of encouraging different perspectives—even about basic terminology and definitions—because the differences represent important ideas and keep the field more inclusive to different perspectives and open to conversations among them (Hesse-Biber & Johnson, 2013). As you consider the use of mixed methods research, you need to recognize that you are now part of these ongoing dialogues and conversations and will likely be called on to offer and explain your opinions.

3. What is the best name for this field? Although the name *mixed methods research* has been well established as the identifier of the field through scholarly publications (e.g., JMMR) and organizations (e.g., Mixed Methods International Research Association [MMIRA]), not all members of the field agree that this is the best name. Some prefer *mixed method* as opposed to *mixed methods* (e.g., Morse & Niehaus, 2009). Others believe that the word *method(s)* in the name is too limiting, opting for the broader term of *mixed research* (e.g., Johnson & Onwuegbuzie, 2004). Others have a preference for explicitly stating *quantitative and qualitative* as part of the name (e.g., Morgan, 2014). As with the continuation of multiple perspectives for definitions, it appears likely that some authors will continue using different terms to name the field. Therefore, you need to thoughtfully consider and explain the term that you use with reference to mixed methods in your research practice.

4. What counts as mixed methods research? Stemming from differences in definitions, a continuing debate is what "counts" as mixed methods research. Scholars writing about mixed methods have raised many questions on this point to be debated. Creswell and Plano Clark (2007) questioned whether a content analysis (where a qualitative data set is analyzed for categories, counted, and then analyzed statistically) is an example of mixed methods research. Johnson and Onwuegbuzie (2004) questioned whether a study that mixes quantitative and qualitative language (e.g., words and numbers in a report) might be considered an example of mixed methods research. Morse and Niehaus (2009) questioned whether the development of a quantitative instrument based on qualitative results is an example of mixed methods research. The different answers found to questions like these are indicative of scholars using different definitions for mixed methods. Do not discount these differences when you encounter them, but keep in mind that they are demonstrating important perspectives that coexist within the field.

These four questions highlight ongoing debates and issues related to defining mixed methods research and the importance such definitions have for the field. They also point to the importance of explicitly articulating and considering how mixed methods research is defined whenever you read about or use mixed methods research. These differing opinions make the field of mixed methods research more complex and challenging but also more interesting, nuanced, and inclusive.

APPLYING DEFINITIONS IN MIXED METHODS RESEARCH PRACTICE

Just as the field continues to consider and debate how to define mixed methods research, you need to explicitly consider how it is being defined whenever you engage in mixed methods research practice as a reader, reviewer, or researcher. This is equally important when reading and reviewing the literature about mixed methods research as when proposing, reporting, or discussing your use of mixed methods research. In Box 3.1, we offer some general advice for applying the concepts of this chapter to your mixed methods research practice.

When reading and reviewing the literature about mixed methods research, it is essential to keep in mind that important variations exist in how scholars define mixed methods research. As you read and evaluate the mixed methods literature,

---

Box 3.1

Advice for Applying Definitions in Mixed Methods Research Practice

Advice for Reading/Reviewing Mixed Methods Studies and Methodological Discussions

- Identify the term(s) that the authors used to name the mixed methods approach.
- Identify the authors' definition for this approach and whether it was stated explicitly or merely implied.
- Note how the authors justified their definition, such as by citing specific references or explaining the reasons for their definition.
- Note what perspectives (i.e., methods, methodology, philosophy, and/or community of research practice) the authors emphasized in the definition.
- Assess the extent to which the authors' terminology and definition reflected one of the prominent perspectives found in the methodological literature.

- Assess the extent to which the authors' definition of mixed methods research aligned with their mixed methods research practice.

Advice for Proposing/Reporting/Discussing Mixed Methods Research

- Choose a definition for mixed methods research that best matches your perspectives.
- Refer to your overall mixed methods approach using a common term (e.g., mixed methods research) so that others can recognize and identify your work.
- Provide the definition for mixed methods research in your writing, and consider including an explanation of why you are using this specific definition.
- Include at least one citation to the literature to support the stated definition.

we advise that you look for the definition (and supporting citations) that the authors have used and recognize that they may have used one of several different perspectives about what is being integrated or mixed in mixed methods research. By identifying the authors' perspective(s), you may better understand the issues they are considering and the ideas they are emphasizing. In addition, we recommend assessing the extent to which the authors' perspectives were supported by the mixed methods literature, explained in the context of the literature about the research topic of interest, and consistent with the overall theoretical or empirical approach used. For example, it would be inconsistent for an author to have defined mixed methods research in terms of mixing philosophical perspectives but then not to have discussed the philosophical foundations for the research study.

It is also important to consider your definition of mixed methods research when you report on the design and conduct of your mixed methods research study. On the one hand, readers who are knowledgeable about mixed methods research will likely be looking for the definition as part of their review because they know that different definitions exist. On the other hand, since mixed methods research is still relatively new, many readers may be unfamiliar with the term and not know what you mean by *mixed methods research*. There are also conflicting and incorrect definitions published in the popular and non-academic literature, so it is possible that some readers will approach your work with incorrect or different ideas about mixed methods research. Therefore, we advise that you carefully define what you mean by *mixed methods* and cite relevant sources (such as those listed in Table 3.1) to support your definition in your scholarly writings and presentations.

CONCLUDING COMMENTS

We conclude the chapter by offering some final summary comments organized by the learning objectives stated at the beginning of the chapter.

- **Understand commonly used terminology for defining mixed methods research.** Scholars engaging with the field of mixed methods research need to decide how to refer to the field. *Mixed methods research* is the most prominent term and therefore the term we selected for use in this book. Other common terms that best capture the essence of the field include *mixed method research, mixed research,* and some combination of *quantitative and qualitative.*
- **Identify the different ways that mixed methods research is defined, and consider the implications of these differences for mixed methods research practice.** The field of mixed methods research has not settled on one single definition for this approach. Most definitions vary in terms of the level at which the integration or mixing of the quantitative and qualitative approaches is thought to occur. The different perspectives view mixing occurring at the levels of methods, methodology, philosophy, and/or research communities. Each of these perspectives has value for thinking about and conducting mixed methods research, and the diversity adds richness to the field. When engaging with the field of mixed methods research, it is important to identify the definition being used and recognize that the definition has an influence on mixed methods research practice.
- **Articulate the definition for mixed methods research that aligns with your perspectives about mixing methods.** When planning and disseminating information about mixed methods research, scholars should provide a definition that fits their perspectives and contexts.

A good strategy is to review the prominent definitions in the field (such as those in Table 3.1), select the definition that conveys the perspective(s) that are consistent with your thinking about mixed methods, and include citations to support your stated definition for your audiences.

APPLICATION QUESTIONS

1. The word cloud pictured in Figure 3.3 was made from the text of the 10 definitions for mixed methods research listed in Table 3.1. The relative size of the words represents their relative frequency within the definitions.
   a. Examine the words in the largest-sized fonts. About which facets is there extensive agreement for defining mixed methods research?
   b. Examine the words in the mid-sized fonts. About which facets is there good agreement for defining mixed methods research?
   c. Examine the words in the smallest-sized fonts. About which facets are there the most differences in perspectives for defining mixed methods research?

2. Examine the definitions in Table 3.1, and decide which definition(s) best align with your perspectives about mixed methods research. Write a statement that articulates the definition that you would use to guide your application of mixed methods research. Explain why you chose this definition among the different possibilities, and discuss how the definition might shape your mixed methods research practice.

3. Locate an example of mixed methods research from your discipline and area of interest. Identify the term(s) that the authors used to identify their use of mixed methods and whether they included an explicit definition. Describe the perspectives you find present in their definition, and critique the clarity and appropriateness of the definition.

4. Pick one of the ongoing issues and debates highlighted in this chapter about mixed methods research terminology and definitions. Discuss your opinion about this issue in terms of how mixed methods research is defined within the field of mixed methods research.

Figure 3.3 Word Cloud of the Text of Ten Definitions of Mixed Methods Research

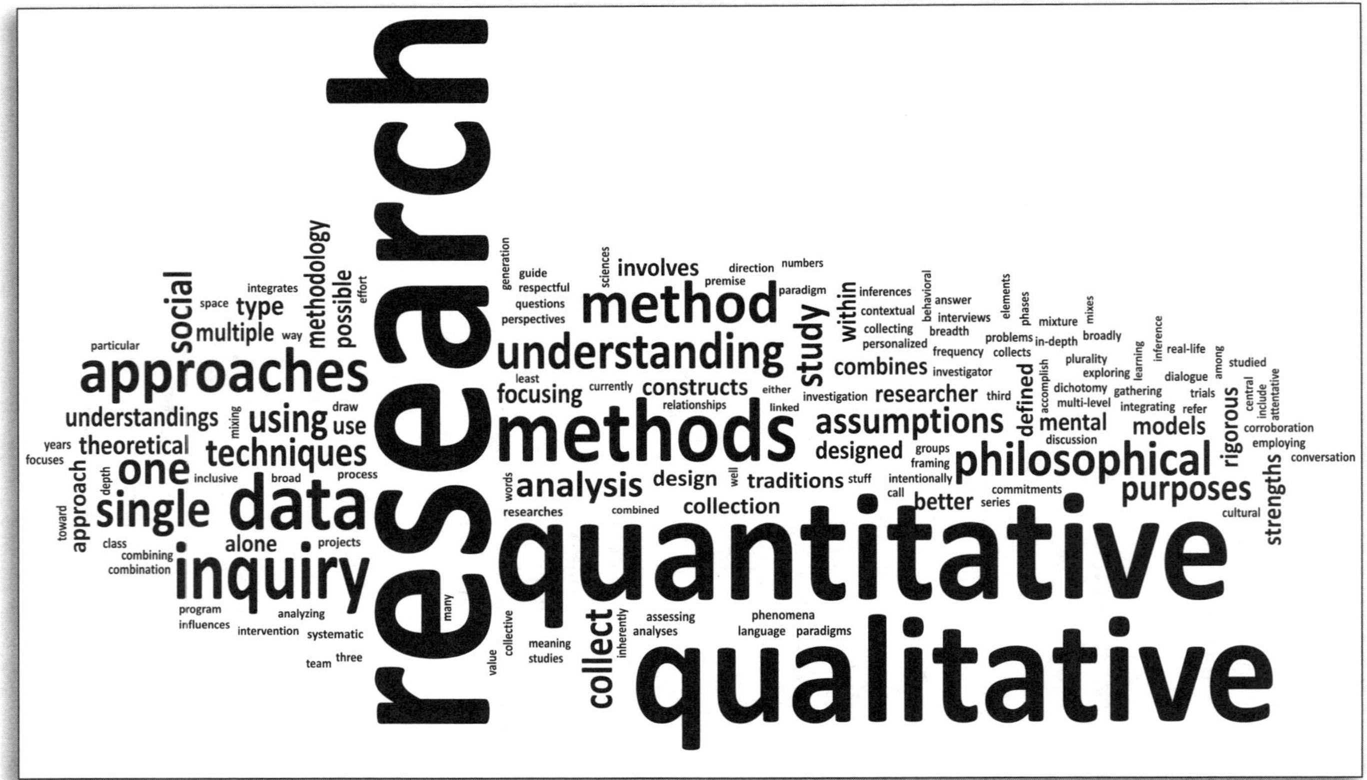

SOURCE: Wordle.net.

KEY RESOURCES

To learn more about the considerations, issues, and debates around defining mixed methods research, we suggest you start with the following resources:

*1. **Johnson, R. B., Onwuegbuzie, A. J., & Turner, L. A. (2007). Toward a definition of mixed methods research.** *Journal of Mixed Methods Research, 1*(2), 112–133.

 • In this article, Johnson and colleagues provided an in-depth historical overview of mixed methods research as well as an analysis of 19 contemporary definitions offered by prominent writers in the field.

*2. **Tashakkori, A., & Creswell, J. W. (2007). The new era of mixed methods [Editorial].** *Journal of Mixed Methods Research, 1*(1), 3–7.

 • In this editorial, which appeared in the debut issue of the JMMR, Tashakkori and Creswell provided the definition of mixed methods research that they used to initiate the journal.

3. **Teddlie, C., & Tashakkori, A. (2003). Major issues and controversies in the use of mixed methods in the social and behavioral sciences. In A. Tashakkori & C. Teddlie (Eds.),** *Handbook of mixed methods in social & behavioral research* **(pp. 3–50). Thousand Oaks, CA: Sage.**

 • In this opening chapter of the first *Handbook of Mixed Methods,* Teddlie and Tashakkori described the many issues and controversies present in the field of mixed methods research, including how it is defined and the language that is used. Most of these issues continue to be discussed and debated today.

* The key resource is available at the following website: http://study.sagepub.com/planoclark.

❧ FOUR ❧

WHY USE MIXED METHODS RESEARCH?

IDENTIFYING RATIONALES FOR MIXING METHODS

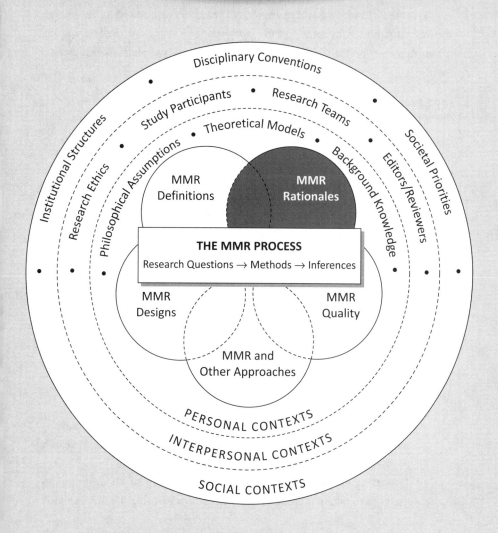

*N*ow that you understand how mixed methods research is defined, a natural next question for you to ask is this: Why use it? Much of the conversation found within the mixed methods literature seeks to answer this question. From the time scholars were first conceptualizing mixed methods research, they have emphasized rationales for why it is useful and appropriate to combine quantitative and qualitative approaches in research practice. There is general consensus in the field that mixed methods should be used when one approach (quantitative or qualitative) is insufficient and both approaches combined can lead to a better understanding of the research purpose. That said, there are also many different ideas about the specific reasons why a better understanding can be achieved by mixing methods. Therefore, you need to be able to identify different rationales for justifying the use of mixed methods as an important consideration for navigating the field of mixed methods research.

LEARNING OBJECTIVES

This chapter aims to provide you with an understanding of rationales for using mixed methods research so you are able to do the following:

- Understand the role of rationales in mixed methods research.
- Identify different possible reasons to justify the use of mixed methods research.
- Consider the appropriateness of a stated rationale within the context of mixed methods research practice.

CHAPTER 4 KEY CONCEPTS

The following key concepts will help you navigate through the main considerations related to identifying mixed methods rationales as they are introduced in this chapter:

- **Mixed methods rationales:** Explicit arguments for and the reasons why the use of mixed methods research is needed to address research problems and purposes.
- **Offsetting strengths and weaknesses:** An argument for using mixed methods to obtain more rigorous conclusions by using the two methods

such that the strengths of the quantitative methods offset the weaknesses of the qualitative methods and vice versa.

- **Triangulation:** An argument for using mixed methods to obtain more valid conclusions about a phenomenon by directly comparing the results obtained from quantitative methods to those obtained from qualitative methods for convergence and divergence.
- **Complementarity:** An argument for using mixed methods to obtain more complete conclusions by using quantitative and qualitative methods to get complementary results about different facets of a phenomenon.
- **Development:** An argument for using mixed methods to develop more effective and refined conclusions by using the results from one method to inform or shape the use of the other method.
- **Social justice rationale:** An argument for using mixed methods to uncover and challenge oppression in society by using quantitative and qualitative methods to best conduct research guided by a social justice perspective.

THE ROLE OF RATIONALES IN THE FIELD OF MIXED METHODS RESEARCH

With the many research approaches available, scholars need sound reasons to justify whichever approach they choose to use within a particular research situation. As a relatively new research approach, the field of mixed methods research has been especially concerned with articulating a set of good reasons that scholars can use to justify their choice to employ mixed methods. Thus, extensive literature has developed around the rationales suitable for mixing methods (Bryman, 2006a; Greene, Caracelli, & Graham, 1989; Johnson & Onwuegbuzie, 2004; Newman, Ridenour, Newman, & DeMarco, 2003). **Mixed methods rationales** are the explicit arguments for and reasons that researchers advance for using mixed methods research to address their research problems and purposes. By delineating a range of appropriate rationales, scholars have worked to legitimize mixed methods research as an approach for which there exists strong arguments in support of its use (as opposed to it being viewed as a fad or something that researchers do on a whim). Due to the importance of such arguments in the field, many of the available definitions of mixed methods research include a reference to its rationale. Looking back at Table 3.1, you can find several definitions that include a broad overall rationale for mixing methods with phrases such as "provides a better understanding" (Creswell & Plano Clark, 2011, p. 5), "for the breadth and depth of understanding and corroboration" (Johnson, Onwuegbuzie, & Turner, 2007, p. 123), and "will accomplish more" (Morgan, 2014, p. xiii).

Rationales for mixing methods continue to be an important methodological content consideration for the field even as it has become more accepted and established. This importance becomes clear when considering the role of rationales within mixed methods research practice. As highlighted in our conceptual framework for mixed methods research and depicted in Figure 4.1, the

Figure 4.1 The Role of Rationales in the Practice of Mixed Methods Research

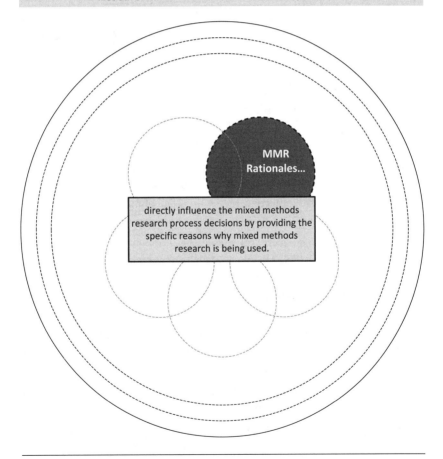

NOTE: MMR = mixed methods research.

mixed methods research process is directly influenced by researchers' rationales for using this approach to research, and the consideration of mixed methods rationales is shaped by the researchers' contexts, such as their personal and disciplinary assumptions about research. As we discussed in Chapter 2, the mixed methods research process is complex, and researchers make many decisions when using mixed methods research. To successfully negotiate this complexity, researchers need sound arguments for why they are integrating methods. The mixed methods rationales serve to guide many of the research process decisions, such as whether to use a concurrent or a sequential mixed methods approach and how to plan for integrating the quantitative and qualitative study components. When mixed methods research is of good quality, there is a clear logic and consistency between the researchers' rationales for mixing and what they actually do in their research practice (O'Cathain, 2010). In some mixed methods projects, researchers find that refined or new rationales emerge while a study is being conducted because of the insights gained from initial results (Bryman, 2006a). Therefore, to understand and assess the research process used in mixed methods studies and to conduct mixed methods research thoughtfully, it is important that you understand that several different reasons for mixing methods may be warranted and that rationales have important implications for how mixed methods research is applied in practice.

MAJOR PERSPECTIVES ABOUT RATIONALES FOR MIXED METHODS RESEARCH

When researchers choose to use mixed methods research, they need to justify why it is an appropriate choice for the particular research problem and purpose of interest. Conceptually, the overall argument advanced for the use of mixed methods research is: One method alone is insufficient to address the study's research problem and purpose, and a combination of quantitative and qualitative methods will result in a better understanding. Although at first glance this provides a strong rationale for the need to mix methods, upon further reflection it also suggests several important questions. In what situations can one argue that one method is insufficient? If all research approaches aim to add to our understanding of issues, then what kinds of "better understandings" can be found from a mixed methods approach? It is the answers to questions like these that the field of mixed methods has attempted to resolve when considering rationales for mixed methods research.

One prominent argument for mixing methods is that different methods have different strengths and weaknesses, and they can be effectively combined to take advantage of these differences (Bryman, 2006a; Johnson & Onwuegbuzie, 2004; Reichardt & Cook, 1979). This argument is sometimes referred to as **offsetting strengths and weaknesses,** where the reason for using mixed methods is to obtain more rigorous conclusions by using the two methods such that the strengths of the quantitative methods offset the weaknesses of the qualitative methods and vice versa. For example, researchers may argue that they need to use quantitative methods with a large representative sample to produce results that can be generalized (a "strength"), but note that those generalized results will lack detail about the particular contexts (a "weakness"). Therefore, in addition they argue for the need to also use qualitative methods with a small, purposeful sample to provide a rich description of context (a "strength") even though those descriptive findings will be limited to a few specific cases (a "weakness"). By thoughtfully combining the two types of methods, the overall argument is that the researchers will obtain and integrate different results that compensate for each other and jointly provide a better understanding of the research problem. We already introduced the basic premise of this rationale in Chapter 1 with Johnson and Turner's (2003) fundamental principle of mixed methods research.

Another important argument for why researchers need to combine quantitative and qualitative research is based on the concept of triangulation. The term *triangulation* originally comes from geometry and surveying and relates to the process of determining the precise location of a point in space based on the measurement of two or more different angles and distances. Qualitative researchers adopted the metaphor of triangulation to describe the process of developing more credible and accurate conclusions by grounding them in multiple perspectives, such as multiple participants, multiple methods (e.g., observations and interviews), multiple theories, or multiple researchers (Denzin, 1978; Lincoln & Guba, 1985). Building on the concept of triangulation from qualitative research, several scholars in the 1970s argued that better (i.e., more valid and more corroborated) understandings can occur in research when one draws conclusions based on the results of *both* quantitative *and* qualitative methods (e.g., Jick, 1979; Reichardt & Cook, 1979). In mixed methods research, **triangulation** is the argument for using mixed methods to obtain more valid conclusions about a phenomenon by directly comparing the results obtained from quantitative methods to those obtained from qualitative methods for convergence and divergence. The argument of triangulation continues to be a common and powerful rationale for mixing methods (Greene et al., 1989; Mertens & Hesse-Biber, 2012). For example, researchers argue for using mixed methods to develop well-validated (i.e., triangulated) conclusions by comparing statistical results obtained from a quantitative survey with thematic results obtained from qualitative interviews. If the results from the different methods agree, researchers can be more confident in what they found, but if any discrepancies occur between the two sets of results then the researchers need to take further steps to try to reconcile why different methods led to different results (Creswell & Plano Clark, 2011; Wagner et al., 2012).

A third prominent rationale for mixing methods is complementarity. **Complementarity** is the argument for using mixed methods to obtain more complete conclusions by using quantitative and qualitative methods to get complementary results about different facets of a phenomenon (Greene et al., 1989). There are many different reasons found in the literature why researchers use complementarity as the basis for their argument. Complementarity occurs when researchers argue for the need to integrate methods to develop a more complete picture by addressing different research questions or research goals (Bryman, 2006a; Morgan, 2014; Reichardt & Cook, 1979; Teddlie & Tashakkori, 2009). For example, researchers may need to integrate qualitative methods to explore a process and complementary quantitative methods to examine outcomes from that process. Another example of complementarity occurs when researchers need quantitative methods to describe general trends about variables and qualitative methods to illustrate the details of those trends. As a final example of complementarity, some researchers argue for the need to use different methods to examine different levels of a system (e.g., quantitative surveys of patients, qualitative focus group interviews with nurses, quantitative measures of clinicians, and qualitative observations of clinics) to develop a more complete and multifaceted understanding. Whereas triangulation is an argument for obtaining more valid conclusions by comparing and contrasting quantitative and qualitative results, complementarity aims to obtain conclusions that are more meaningful and complete by using the two methods to get results that enhance coverage and clarify and/or supplement each other to address the complexity of a topic.

When researchers' rationales for mixing methods include triangulation and complementarity, they most often choose to use concurrent timing for the quantitative and qualitative components of their mixed methods studies. Alternatively, when researchers have a rationale of development, they often choose to use sequential timing in their mixed methods studies

(Creswell & Plano Clark, 2011; Greene, 2007). **Development** is the argument for using mixed methods to develop more effective and refined conclusions by using the results from one method (quantitative or qualitative) to inform or shape the use of the other method (qualitative or quantitative) (Greene et al., 1989). There are many possible reasons why researchers' rationales include development. For example, researchers who want to understand why certain factors predict students' involvement at school might argue for the need to quantitatively assess significant predictors and then use the quantitative results to develop a qualitative follow-up exploration aimed at explaining why certain factors were significant. This is an example of development because the results from the quantitative methods shape the use of the qualitative methods. Another example of development is researchers needing to obtain qualitative findings about a topic in order to use those qualitative findings to inform the development of a new instrument, material, or program, which is then tested quantitatively. Researchers also argue development when they need to use the results of one method to inform the sampling plan for the other method, such as identifying extreme results using quantitative methods and then sampling the extreme cases for further exploration using qualitative methods.

Another rationale for mixing methods that is receiving increased attention in the field might best be called a social justice rationale. A **social justice rationale** is an argument for mixing methods to uncover and challenge oppression in society by using quantitative and qualitative methods to best conduct research guided by a social justice perspective. In contrast to the other rationales we have discussed that emphasize methodological considerations, a social justice rationale has as much or more to do with ideology and researchers' values (Caracelli & Greene, 1997). A social justice rationale for mixed methods will likely emphasize the need to mix quantitative and qualitative methods as the best way to involve participants from the community as research partners, to empower participants, to expose injustices, to raise awareness of multiple stakeholder groups, and to bring about transformations in society (Mertens, 2003; Onwuegbuzie & Frels, 2013). For example, researchers may argue for using quantitative methods to document the existence of unequal treatment of people and qualitative methods to give voice to those who have been marginalized. Another example would be researchers arguing for the need to mix methods because the different methods will produce results that are viewed as credible to the different relevant stakeholder groups (such as qualitative narrative findings being viewed as more credible by community partners and quantitative statistical results being viewed as more credible by policy makers).

Although offsetting strengths and weaknesses, triangulation, complementarity, development, and social justice rationales encompass prominent reasons for mixing methods, they are not the only rationales discussed in the literature. Additional perspectives exist, such as needing to integrate methods to include diverse perspectives, to search for paradox and contradictions among the results of different methods, and to obtain results that are useful or credible for audiences (Bryman, 2006a; Greene et al., 1989; Teddlie & Tashakkori, 2009). The key to understanding mixed methods rationales is that researchers need to consider and state sound arguments for why mixed methods is warranted and to guide their mixed methods research practice decisions. Oftentimes, there are several possible rationales and researchers advance either one or several rationales to justify their use of this approach. The diverse nature of the many rationales can be confusing when researchers first encounter this approach, but the fact that many possible rationales have been noted in the mixed methods literature speaks to the overall complexity and utility of mixed methods research.

EXAMPLES OF RATIONALES FOR MIXED METHODS RESEARCH

Due to the variety of possible rationales for mixing methods, there are many different examples found within the literature. Methodologists writing about mixed methods have focused on delineating sets of reasons to guide researchers' choices and researchers tend to offer the specific rationale that has guided their decisions in planning and conducting a specific mixed methods research study. We examine these two different approaches to mixed methods rationales in the following sections.

Rationales From the Methodological Literature

A wide array of perspectives about the rationales for mixing methods occurs within the mixed methods methodological literature. Although there are writings that focus on a single rationale (such as triangulation), many of the available methodological writings have attempted to develop and describe sets of the different reasons that are suitable for arguing for mixed methods research. These sets of options are often referred to as *typologies* in the mixed methods literature. We have listed examples of six such typologies of mixed methods rationales in Table 4.1. For each typology, we list the different reasons along with brief descriptions of the

Table 4.1 Six Typologies of Rationales for Using Mixed Methods Research

Authors	Mixed Methods Research Rationales	Comments
Reichardt and Cook (1979)	1. **Multiple purposes** (to examine both process and outcomes) 2. **Each method-type building upon the other** (to use the knowledge gained from one method to benefit and complement the other) 3. **Triangulation through converging operations** (to correct for biases present in each method)	This typology: • is provided by authors writing in the context of evaluation. • is one of the earliest sets of rationales found in the field.
Greene, Caracelli, and Graham (1989)	1. **Triangulation** (to increase the validity of results by converging and corroborating results from the different methods) 2. **Complementarity** (to increase the interpretability and meaningfulness of results by elaborating, enhancing, illustrating, and clarifying the results from one method with the results from the other method) 3. **Development** (to increase the validity of results by using the results from one method to help inform the sampling, measurement, and implementation of the other method) 4. **Initiation** (to increase the breadth and depth of results and interpretations by discovering paradox and contradiction, advancing new perspectives of frameworks, and recasting questions or results from one method with questions or results from the other method)	This typology: • is provided by authors writing in the context of evaluation. • was derived theoretically and then applied in a review of 57 published mixed methods evaluation studies. • is still cited extensively 25 years after publication.

	5. **Expansion** (to increase the scope of a study by using different methods for different study components)
Collins, Onwuegbuzie, and Sutton (2006)	1. **Participant enrichment** (to combine methods to optimize the study sample by improving recruitment, determining inclusion criteria, or understanding participants' reactions to the study) 2. **Instrument fidelity** (to combine methods to maximize the appropriateness and utility of data collection instruments and protocols) 3. **Treatment integrity** (to combine methods to assess the fidelity and context of interventions, treatments, and programs) 4. **Significance enhancement** (to combine methods to enhance interpretations of data, analyses, and results)	This typology: • is provided by authors writing in the context of special education. • was derived from a content analysis of empirical studies and methodological discussions. • emphasizes a few broad reasons for mixing methods.

(Continued)

Table 4.1 (Continued)

Authors	Mixed Methods Research Rationales	Comments
Bryman (2006a)	1. **Triangulation or greater validity** (to combine quantitative and qualitative research to corroborate findings) 2. **Offset** (to offset the weaknesses and draw on the strengths associated with both quantitative and qualitative research) 3. **Completeness** (to bring together a more comprehensive account of the study topic) 4. **Process and structure** (to use quantitative research to provide an account of structures in social life and qualitative research to provide a sense of process) 5. **Different research questions** (to use quantitative and qualitative research to answer different research questions) 6. **Explanation** (to use one method to help explain findings generated by the other) 7. **Unexpected results** (to understand surprising results from one method by employing the other method) 8. **Instrument development** (to use qualitative research to inform the development of questionnaire and scale items) 9. **Sampling** (to use one approach to facilitate the sampling of respondents or cases for the other approach)	This typology: • is provided by an author writing in the context of the social sciences. • was derived empirically from the reasons provided by authors in 232 published social science studies. • emphasizes many specific reasons for mixing methods.

10. **Credibility** (to enhance the integrity of findings by employing both approaches)

11. **Context** (to provide contextual understanding from qualitative research with broad relationships or generalizable results from quantitative research)

12. **Illustration** (to use qualitative data to illustrate quantitative results)

13. **Utility or improving the usefulness of findings** (to develop results that are more useful to practitioners and others)

14. **Confirm and discover** (to use qualitative research to generate hypotheses and quantitative research to test them)

15. **Diversity of views** (to combine the researchers' perspectives as found in selected variables through quantitative research with participants' perspectives as found in emergent meanings through qualitative research)

16. **Enhancement or building upon quantitative and qualitative findings** (to augment one type of findings with data from the other research approach)

(Continued)

Table 4.1 (Continued)

Authors	Mixed Methods Research Rationales	Comments
Teddlie and Tashakkori (2009)	1. **Addressing confirmatory and exploratory questions** (to use different methods to address questions that call to both verify and generate theory in the same study) 2. **Providing stronger inferences** (to develop better conclusions by combining methods so that they offset the disadvantages that each method has on its own) 3. **Providing opportunity for greater assortment of divergent views** (to use different methods to uncover divergent results and include diverse perspectives and voices)	This typology: • is provided by authors writing in the context of social and behavioral research. • emphasizes a few broad reasons for mixing methods.
Morgan (2014)	1. **Convergent findings** (to use both methods to address the same research question to produce greater certainty in the conclusions) 2. **Additional coverage** (to use the strengths of different methods to best achieve different goals within the study) 3. **Sequential contributions** (to enhance the effectiveness of one method with the other method by using what is learned from one method to inform the other)	This typology: • is provided by an author writing in the context of sociology and the health sciences. • emphasizes a few broad reasons for mixing methods.

arguments behind the reasons. We also provide our comments, including the authors' approach to developing the typology and any notable contexts. As the table illustrates, methodologists have approached the development of such typologies in different ways, such as from a theoretical perspective (e.g., Greene et al., 1989) or by examining what researchers actually state in their study reports (e.g., Bryman, 2006a). The typologies also range from many detailed reasons to a few broad reasons and represent several different disciplinary contexts. We purposefully included the different typologies to introduce you to the range of perspectives found in the field. In addition, these six typologies represent the most cited reasons for mixing methods and are therefore the reasons you are most likely to encounter in your own research practice when reading about mixed methods, reviewing mixed methods studies, or conceptualizing your own use of mixed methods research.

Rationales Used in Mixed Methods Research Studies

Researchers who choose to use mixed methods research in their studies do so for all the different types of reasons listed in Table 4.1. With so many different reasons possible, it is recommended that researchers carefully consider and clearly report their rationales within the reports of their mixed methods research studies (O'Cathain, 2010). If no rationale is provided, then readers are unclear why mixed methods is being used and are left to conclude that both the researchers and reviewers were unaware of the importance of this methodological consideration for mixed methods research. In these cases, the researchers simply report the details of their research process without explaining *why* they decided to use mixed methods in the first place.

When researchers incorporate statements of their rationales in reports of their mixed methods studies, they tend to use one of several different approaches. One common approach is when researchers provide a justification for using a second method in addition to a "usual" method. This type of rationale is often used for research problems where the research is usually done in a certain way (quantitative or qualitative). For example, Quan-Haase (2007) justified the complementary use of qualitative focus groups in addition to a typical quantitative survey to achieve a more complete description of Canadian university students' modes of communication in the following way:

These qualitative [focus group] data enriched the survey results and provided a deeper understanding of the social context of Internet use compared with what would be obtained through the survey alone. (p. 673)

In a similar fashion, Evans, Belyea, Coon, and Ume (2012) provided the following reason for including a complementary quantitative component in addition to their qualitative case study approach for developing a more complete description of the daily lives of Mexican American caregivers:

> The addition of a simultaneous, complementary, quantitatively driven, variable-oriented component enables integrated naturalistic and statistical examination of patterns within- and across-cases, and facilitates the drawing of inferences during the analytic and interpretive phases of the study. (p. 444)

Although justifying the reason for a second method is one useful strategy, many stated rationales go further by addressing the reason for using an overall mixed methods approach (not just the reason for the additional method). For example, in their health services research study, Krein et al. (2008) justified the use of mixed methods to better examine the complexity of their topic by stating the following:

> We combined quantitative and qualitative data to allow for a more detailed analysis of the complex phenomena that are inherent in the delivery of healthcare services. (pp. 933–934)

Another example of offering an overall justification for the use of mixed methods in terms of its completeness and utility comes from Ellis, Marsh, and Craven's (2009) evaluation study of a peer support program for Australian high school students. These authors argued the following:

> A combination of quantitative and qualitative methods were used in recognition of recent developments which demonstrate that mixed methods studies can help elucidate various aspects of the phenomenon under investigation, providing a more holistic understanding of it, and resulting in better-informed recommendations (Davies 2000; Marsh et al. 2005b; Steckler et al. 1992). (p. 56)

Hodgkin (2008), working from a feminist stance, provided a social justice rationale for her use of mixed methods to study gender inequities related to social capital. Her argument was centered on "the power of the mixed methods approach to highlight gender inequality" (p. 297). She described several ways in which the use of mixed methods could augment a feminist research approach and concluded with the following:

> Quantitative and qualitative methods can be used together to give a more powerful voice to women's experiences. (p. 299)

An effective approach to stating the rationale is to provide several reasons for mixing methods. Farmer and Knapp (2008) provided three reasons for why they mixed methods in their sequential mixed methods study of the interpretive programs at a U.S. historical site. Note how they refer to the rationales of offsetting weaknesses, development, and complementarity in the following passage:

> The rationale for using the current design was threefold. First, the researchers wanted to comprehend and explore phenomenon from the interpretive experience via multiple approaches, using quantitative and qualitative data, to offset the limitations for using only one medium in analyzing the experience. Second, by using different methods throughout the study, one method was used to inform the construction and implementation of the proceeding method. Finally, the use of mixed methods allowed for a more comprehensive understanding regarding the interpretive experience. (p. 342)

A final example of how researchers justify the use of mixed methods is when researchers provide a rationale for their specific mixed methods design. Jang, McDougall, Pollon, Herbert, and Russell (2008) used this approach when stating complementarity as the rationale for their concurrent mixed methods design to gain insight into how schools facing challenging circumstances experience success from the perspective of principals, teachers, parents, and students:

> This concurrent mixed methods design was to serve the complementarity function in that the general description of school improvement from the survey was enriched, elaborated, and clarified with contextually specific accounts of school success from interviews involving multiple perspectives. (p. 226)

Similarly, Jones-Harris (2010) justified the use of a sequential design for the reason of development in her study to describe and measure how chiropractors in the United Kingdom perceive their role within the primary healthcare setting. She wrote the following:

> The research implemented a sequential study of exploratory design. . . . Such use of the results from a qualitative study to inform a survey is said to enhance the sensitivity and accuracy of the survey questions [22]. The design can also be used to generalise qualitative findings to different samples [23] as well as to determine the distribution of a phenomenon within a chosen population [24]. (p. 3)

The examples provided in this section demonstrate several different strategies that researchers use to state their rationale to indicate their argument for integrating quantitative and qualitative methods. You can use these examples as models for both recognizing the rationales you encounter when reading about mixed methods and crafting statements of rationale when you conceptualize and design your own mixed methods research projects.

ISSUES AND DEBATES ABOUT RATIONALES

Rationales for mixing methods are an important consideration within the mixed methods literature and mixed methods research practice. Across the field, there is extensive consensus regarding the importance of justifying one's use of mixed methods research and that strong arguments for using mixed methods are built from the need to develop better understandings by combining methods. Despite the consensus, there are still issues and debates among the different perspectives that exist within the field about this methodological consideration, often arising from differences in scholars' personal, interpersonal, and social contexts. Here, we briefly introduce three issues that have been raised about rationales for mixing methods.

1. Do rationales for mixing methods necessarily align with mixed methods research practice? The mixed methods literature advocates that researchers clearly articulate a defensible rationale to justify mixing methods. In fact, the articulation of a sound rationale is included as a major criterion in several writings about quality in mixed methods research (Heyvaert, Hannes, Maes, & Onghena, 2013). (We will discuss quality considerations further in Chapter 7.) Despite its importance, reviews of researchers' use of mixed methods research have revealed that authors of mixed methods studies often do not explicitly state a rationale in their study reports (Bryman, 2006a; Plano Clark et al., 2014). Interestingly, Bryman (2006a) found that even when authors stated a rationale, it often did not match their actual use of mixed methods research in the study. These observations suggest that issues continue to exist around justifying mixed methods research. When conducting mixed methods research, you need to carefully consider your rationale at the start of a study and be aware that the reasons may expand and/or evolve as the study is conducted, and if that happens, you should also critically review and report these changes.

2. Is the argument of triangulating quantitative and qualitative methods for studying a single phenomenon viable? Although triangulation is one of the most often cited rationales for mixing methods (Bryman, 2006a), the premise of this argument is not without its own issues and debates. Many alternative perspectives exist about triangulation as a reason for mixing methods (Mertens & Hesse-Biber, 2012). These perspectives include thinking of it as an argument for directly comparing results from different methods and assessing the extent of agreement to achieve valid conclusions, for comparing results to uncover disagreements that can lead to more insightful conclusions, or for putting the results from different methods in dialogue with each other for greater insights and more nuanced conclusions. Although many of these perspectives arise from different interpretations of the meaning of triangulation, Sale, Lohfeld, and Brazil (2002) questioned the basic premise of this rationale. They argued that triangulation is "not a viable option" (p. 49) because quantitative methods can *never* study the same phenomenon as qualitative methods due to the fundamental differences in the assumptions behind these methods. They suggested that the only viable rationale for mixing methods is the argument to study multiple related, but different, phenomena. You should remember the existence of these vastly different viewpoints whenever you encounter the use of triangulation in the context of mixed methods research.

3. Is the argument of offsetting strengths and weaknesses misguided? Since the earliest writings about mixing methods, many scholars have argued that an appropriate rationale is built on the notion that quantitative and qualitative methods have strengths and weaknesses that can be combined in ways so that one method's weaknesses are offset by the other's strengths (Johnson & Turner, 2003). However, Sandelowski (2012) raised concerns about the soundness of this offsetting rationale. She argued that although different methods have different defining attributes, they do not have inherent strengths and weaknesses. She noted that to assess a strength or a weakness, one must first determine the parameter for making comparisons (e.g., authenticity, freedom, transparency, objectivity, or feasibility) and a judgment as to what constitutes a strength and weakness in terms of that parameter. These judgments can only be determined within the context of a particular research situation, which means that what is a weakness in one study may be a strength in another. Therefore, she urged mixed methods researchers to abandon the offsetting strengths and weaknesses rationale and instead argued for mixing methods based on the need for the different types of information generated by the different methods to address a study's purpose. If you choose to use this rationale, you should at least be very explicit about how you define a strength and a weakness and the assumptions that form the basis of those opinions.

These three questions highlight important issues and debates related to rationales for mixed methods research. They also point to the importance of scholars explicitly considering and articulating their rationale for mixing methods in their research practice, and the need to consider multiple possible rationales. The many different reasons for mixing methods, along with different perspectives about some of these reasons, highlight the complex and diverse nature of mixed methods research.

APPLYING RATIONALES IN MIXED METHODS RESEARCH PRACTICE

Mixed methods scholars have devoted extensive attention to developing many possible arguments for why researchers should choose to use mixed methods research. This means that it is important to consider rationales when engaged in all forms of mixed methods research practice. Rationales are discussed throughout the methodological literature and are a critical component in the planning, conducting, and reporting of mixed methods studies. Box 4.1 includes advice for applying the concepts of this chapter when reading about, reviewing, or conducting mixed methods research.

Box 4.1

Advice for Applying Rationales in Mixed Methods Research Practice

Advice for Reading/Reviewing Mixed Methods Studies and Methodological Discussions

- Identify the authors' argument for using mixed methods research, recognizing that there could be more than one reason.
- Note whether the authors' rationale was stated explicitly or merely implied.
- Note whether the provided rationale reflected one or more of the prominent reasons discussed in the methodological literature (e.g., offsetting strengths and weaknesses, triangulation, complementarity, development, and social justice).
- Note how the authors justified and explained their rationale, such as by citing references to the mixed methods literature.
- Assess the extent to which the authors' rationale provided a compelling and sound argument for the use of mixed methods research.
- Assess the extent to which the authors' rationale for mixing methods aligned with their discussion about or use of mixed methods research.

Advice for Proposing/Reporting/Discussing Mixed Methods Research

- Thoughtfully consider your rationale for using mixed methods research in light of the many possible reasons discussed in the mixed methods literature.
- Identify your overall rationale for mixing methods, noting that this rationale may include multiple reasons.
- Articulate an explicit argument for why you choose to use mixed methods research.
- Name the rationales that make up your argument using terminology advanced in the mixed methods literature.
- Include at least one citation to the literature to support your chosen rationale(s).

(Continued)

(Continued)

- Consider your rationale as you make decisions about the mixed methods research process so that your procedures and rationale align with each other.
- Continue to attend to your rationale throughout your mixed methods research process because your reasons for mixing methods may continue to refine or expand.

When reading and reviewing mixed methods literature, it is important to keep in mind that there are several different reasons why scholars write about and use mixed methods research. As you read and evaluate mixed methods literature, look for explicit arguments why mixed methods research is needed in a specific research situation, and recognize that the authors may have several reasons for their use of mixed methods. By identifying the rationale in research studies, you can better understand why the researchers used mixed methods, which should have directly informed decisions about the mixed methods research process. Therefore, it is important to not only assess the extent to which researchers provided and justified sound rationales for using mixed methods but to also assess the extent to which the mixed methods research process was consistent with the stated rationale. For example, it would be inconsistent for researchers to have argued for the use of mixed methods research for development reasons but then implemented the quantitative and qualitative study components at the same time so that there was no opportunity for the results of one method to inform the other method.

It is also important to consider the rationale for mixed methods research when designing and reporting your own mixed methods research study. Readers who are unfamiliar with mixed methods research will benefit from a clear statement of your reasons for using this approach. Likewise, readers who are familiar with mixed methods research will expect to learn the specific reasons for mixing methods in the project among the many possible reasons. There are many diverse reasons for mixing methods, and we recommend that you provide specific reasons related to your mixed methods design in addition to your general overall rationale for integrating methods. By fully explaining your reasons for mixing methods, readers will be in a better position to understand and evaluate the mixed methods research process in terms of your stated rationales for mixing methods.

CONCLUDING COMMENTS

We conclude the chapter by offering some final summary comments organized by the learning objectives stated at the beginning of the chapter.

- **Understand the role of rationales in mixed methods research.** Rationales are the explicit arguments that explain why scholars choose to use mixed methods research. Mixed methods rationales provide the justification for using this approach and also provide the specific reasons that shape many mixed methods research process decisions. The overall reason to choose to mix methods is that the integration of the quantitative and qualitative methods will lead to better understandings than would be obtained by using only one method.

- **Identify different possible reasons to justify the use of mixed methods research.** There are many sound reasons that have been advanced to argue for the use of mixed methods research, including offsetting strengths and weaknesses, triangulation, complementarity, development, and social justice rationales. Due to the range of possible reasons, scholars have developed various typologies that attempt to organize and classify the many available rationales. These differences highlight a variety of ways that better understandings can result from the integration of quantitative and qualitative methods.

- **Consider the appropriateness of a stated rationale within the context of mixed methods research practice.** When reading, reviewing, proposing, or conducting mixed methods research, the mixed methods rationale is an important consideration. The rationale should build on the reasons discussed in the mixed methods literature, be explicitly articulated, and be supported by references to the literature. In addition, the rationale should clearly align with the use of mixed methods within a research study so that however this study unfolds, it clearly serves to address the stated reasons for mixing methods.

APPLICATION QUESTIONS

1. Locate an example of a mixed methods research study in your area of interest, and identify the authors' rationale for using mixed methods in this example. Discuss how the authors conveyed their rationale

including whether it was stated explicitly and what citations they used to support the rationale. What is your assessment of the soundness of the argument that the authors made?

2. Locate an example of a mixed methods research study in your area of interest. Based on the authors' argument for the study and what they did during the study, classify their reason(s) for mixing methods using two different typologies described in Table 4.1. Explain each of your classification decisions.

3. Examine the six typologies of rationales in Table 4.1, and select one typology that aligns well with your own approach to thinking about mixed methods research. Using the reasons included in that typology, describe three different possible rationales for using mixed methods research to study a problem of interest to you and explain why each of these rationales could be appropriate.

4. Pick one of the ongoing issues and debates about rationales for mixed methods highlighted in this chapter. State why you selected that issue and discuss your reactions to this issue in terms of why mixed methods research is used. Explain the reasons for your opinion and the implications that it may have for how you read, review, or conduct mixed methods research.

KEY RESOURCES

To learn more about the considerations, issues, and debates around rationales for using mixed methods research, we suggest you start with the following resources:

*1. Greene, J. C., Caracelli, V. J., & Graham, W. F. (1989). Toward a conceptual framework for mixed-method evaluation designs. *Educational Evaluation and Policy Analysis, 11*(3), 255–274.

- In this article, Greene and colleagues examined theoretical and empirical writings in evaluation to advance a typology of five broad rationales for mixing methods. These five purposes are still frequently used and cited across a wide range of disciplines.

*2. Bryman, A. (2006). Integrating quantitative and qualitative research: How is it done? *Qualitative Research, 6*(1), 97–113.

- In this article, Bryman reported a review of the prevalence of the rationales stated and used in empirical mixed methods studies published in the social sciences. He examined the five broad rationales developed by Greene and colleagues (1989) and advanced a list of 16 more-specific rationales found in published mixed methods studies.

3. **Sandelowski, M. (2012). The weakness of the strong/weak comparison of modes of inquiry [Editorial].** *Research in Nursing & Health, 35,* 325–327.

- In this editorial, Sandelowski raised concerns about the common discourse in the mixed methods literature that argues for the use of mixed methods for the reason of combining to offset the strengths and weaknesses of quantitative and qualitative methods.

* The key resource is available at the following website: http://study.sagepub.com/planoclark.

❖ FIVE ❖

HOW TO USE MIXED METHODS RESEARCH?

UNDERSTANDING THE BASIC MIXED METHODS DESIGNS

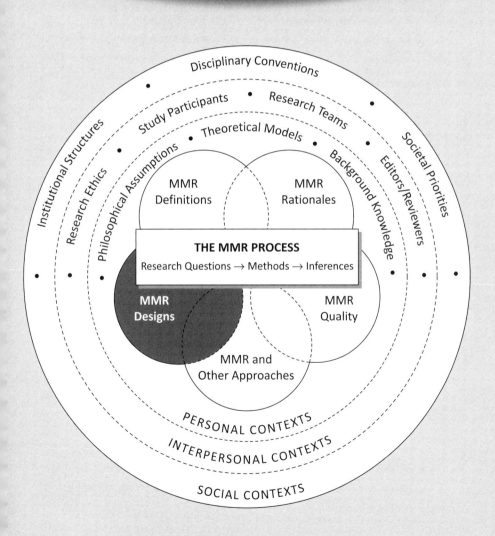

Now that we have introduced you to different rationales for justifying the use of mixed methods research, you may wonder how these decisions relate to the choice of mixed methods designs that guide the mixed methods research process. As we have shown in Chapter 4, different rationales call for different ways of integrating quantitative and qualitative methods in a mixed methods study. Such methods' integration has an underlying logic that reflects how quantitative and qualitative data are collected and analyzed within a specific mixed methods design. Multiple perspectives exist on the type and number of mixed methods research designs and related typologies as well as their role in mixed methods research practice. In this chapter, we describe different perspectives on mixed methods designs and introduce three basic mixed methods designs used in most mixed methods studies to help you understand and navigate this important aspect of the mixed methods research process.

LEARNING OBJECTIVES

This chapter aims to describe mixed methods research designs and how they are used in mixed methods research so you are able to do the following:

- Understand different perspectives about designs for mixed methods research.
- Describe three basic mixed methods designs and their underlying logic.
- Understand how the basic mixed methods designs are applied in research practice.

CHAPTER 5 KEY CONCEPTS

The following key concepts will help you navigate through the main considerations related to understanding mixed methods research designs as they are introduced in this chapter:

- **Mixed methods design:** A research design in which researchers mix quantitative and qualitative methods in specific ways to address a research purpose.

- **Design typology:** A set of different possible mixed methods designs that attempts to convey the range of design options available for the use of mixed methods research.
- **Procedural diagram:** A figure or visual that depicts the flow of the research activities in a mixed methods study.
- **Mixed methods design logic:** A set of decisions about timing, integration, and priority of quantitative and qualitative methods that researchers have to make when designing a mixed methods study.
- **Strand:** A component of a mixed methods study that encompasses the basic process of conducting quantitative or qualitative research: posing a question, collecting and analyzing data, and interpreting results.
- **Concurrent Quan + Qual design:** A mixed methods design in which researchers implement the quantitative and qualitative strands concurrently or independent from each other with the purpose of comparing or merging quantitative and qualitative results to produce more complete and validated conclusions.
- **Sequential Quan → Qual design:** A mixed methods design in which researchers implement the quantitative and qualitative strands in sequence with the purpose of using follow-up qualitative data to elaborate, explain, or confirm initial quantitative results.
- **Sequential Qual → Quan design:** A mixed methods design in which researchers implement the qualitative and quantitative strands in sequence with the purpose of using follow-up quantitative data to generalize, test, or confirm initial qualitative results.

THE ROLE OF DESIGNS IN
THE FIELD OF MIXED METHODS RESEARCH

Mixed methods designs play an important role in how researchers approach the mixed methods research process. We define a **mixed methods design** as a research design in which researchers mix quantitative and qualitative methods in specific ways to address a research purpose. A mixed methods design serves as a framework for researchers to organize their thought process about the order and the manner of how the quantitative and qualitative components are implemented in a mixed methods study process. Therefore, choosing an appropriate design is a key methodological consideration for the mixed methods research process, because a study design guides researchers' decisions related to collecting, analyzing, and integrating quantitative and qualitative data to provide the answers to the posed research questions. Additionally, choosing an appropriate design is useful because it helps "set the logic" by which researchers make interpretations of the quantitative and qualitative results and develop inferences grounded in these conclusions (Creswell & Plano Clark, 2011, p. 53).

The field of mixed methods research abounds in the number and types of mixed methods designs, making the field particularly complex to navigate. Reportedly, the names and types of mixed methods designs "have multiplied over the years" (Creswell, 2015, p. 58). There are many designs to choose from, and often the same design is referred to by different names throughout the mixed methods literature. Despite this variety, most mixed methods studies make use of the same basic mixed methods designs. These basic designs provide an underlying logic for integrating the quantitative and qualitative components during a study process when proceeding from research questions to methods and then to inferences.

Understanding the logic for mixed methods designs and the decisions researchers make about selecting a specific design is a critical aspect of your successful engagement with the practice of mixed methods research. As highlighted in our conceptual framework for mixed methods research and depicted in Figure 5.1, the mixed methods research process is directly influenced by how researchers approach the design of a mixed methods study and what underlying logic they choose to frame the mixed methods research process within a specific design. These decisions are shaped by other mixed methods research content considerations (e.g., the rationale for using mixed methods research) and the influences of the many factors that form researchers' personal, interpersonal, and social contexts.

MAJOR PERSPECTIVES ABOUT DESIGNS FOR MIXED METHODS RESEARCH

Many perspectives exist about the nature and types of mixed methods designs in the mixed methods literature. As we noted in Chapter 3, the idea of integrating quantitative and qualitative methods in a mixed methods

Figure 5.1 The Role of Mixed Methods Designs in the Practice of Mixed Methods Research

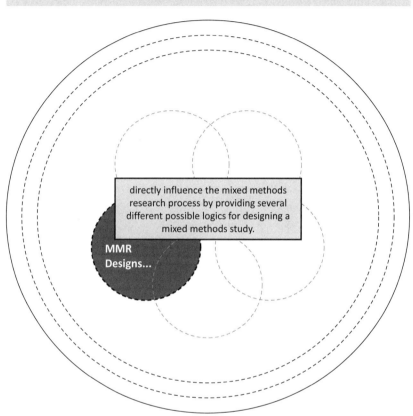

directly influence the mixed methods research process by providing several different possible logics for designing a mixed methods study.

MMR Designs...

NOTE: MMR = mixed methods research.

study is emphasized in many definitions of mixed methods research. For a mixed methods study to be "truly mixed," integration of the quantitative and qualitative methods should occur at different stages in a study process (Teddlie & Tashakkori, 2009, p. 142). This focus on methods' integration is at the core of the current conceptualizations of mixed methods research. It also guides the existing discussions about what constitutes a mixed methods design, how to define and classify different mixed methods designs, and how to visually present the mixed methods procedures used in a study.

Nature of Mixed Methods Designs

Teddlie and Tashakkori (2009) suggested distinguishing between *truly mixed designs* and *quasi-mixed designs*. The latter are the designs where researchers collect and analyze both quantitative and qualitative data but make no attempt to meaningfully mix the methods or results to answer a study's research questions. In a truly mixed methods design study, researchers mix quantitative and qualitative methods to generate inferences grounded in both sets of results. This distinction is very important to help you navigate the existing body of published empirical studies that used both quantitative and qualitative approaches and understand the value added by mixing methods in truly mixed methods designs.

Mixed methods scholars also suggested thinking about mixed methods designs as *fixed* and *emergent* designs (Creswell & Plano Clark, 2011; Morse & Niehaus, 2009). Because mixed methods designs include at least one quantitative and one qualitative component, researchers may plan all components during the study conceptualization and design stage from the start of the study, thus making the design fixed. In contrast, researchers may decide to add a complementary component during the conduct of the study and thus have a mixed methods design emerge. Emergent mixed methods designs are useful when a single employed method (quantitative or qualitative) does not yield the necessary information or results in unexpected findings. In these situations, researchers may determine that there is an emergent need to add a second method (qualitative or quantitative) to augment the initial method in order to fully address the study's intent. In reality, some mixed methods designs originally planned as fixed designs may become emergent designs when researchers decide to add an additional quantitative or qualitative component to address unexpected results or to probe further into the issue.

Approaches to Designs

In addition to the different perspectives about the nature of mixed methods designs, different perspectives exist on the types of mixed methods designs and how researchers should approach designing a mixed methods study. The two distinct approaches to mixed methods designs are typology-based and dynamic. Within a *typology-based approach,* scholars classify mixed methods designs based on some common methodological characteristics and procedural features—thus, creating mixed methods design typologies. Within the context of mixed methods research, a **design typology** is defined as a set of different possible mixed methods designs that attempts to convey the range of design options available. Teddlie and Tashakkori (2009) argued that mixed methods design typologies or prototypes "provide a variety of paths, or ideal design types, that may be chosen to accomplish the goals of the study" (p. 139). Using a typology-based approach, researchers can select a particular mixed methods design from a set of possible options and adapt it to the specific purposes of their study. Many different mixed methods design typologies can be found in the mixed methods literature (e.g., Creswell & Plano Clark, 2011; Greene, 2007; Greene, Caracelli, & Graham, 1989; Guest, 2013; Leech & Onwuegbuzie, 2009; Morgan, 2014; Morse & Niehaus, 2009; Sandelowski, 2000; Teddlie & Tashakkori, 2009).

We listed examples of five mixed methods design typologies in Table 5.1. We purposefully included these typologies because they are often cited in the mixed methods literature, and you may encounter them in your mixed methods research practice. For each typology, we listed the names of the different designs that make up the typology and their characteristics related to timing, mixing, and priority of the quantitative and qualitative methods in a study. We also provided our comments about each typology, including the disciplinary contexts and the authors' approach to developing the typology. As you examine the different mixed methods designs across the typologies, you will likely notice some similarities and some differences in the designs. For example, some designs are named in terms of their purpose (e.g., convergence or exploratory), others in terms of the relationship between the methods (e.g., parallel or sequential), and others in terms of the role for the quantitative or qualitative methods (e.g., drive the design or follow-up). Despite the observed differences in the designs' names and the methodological characteristics used to classify these designs, these typologies have many common features and highlight common design elements that make mixed methods designs distinct and different from other quantitative and qualitative designs. You can use the information in the table to help recognize design names commonly used in the mixed methods literature, note their major characteristics, as well as to identify the primary source for learning more about any one specific mixed methods design.

Table 5.1 Typologies of Mixed Methods Designs

Typologies (Authors)	Mixed Methods Designs	Typical Design Characteristics	Comments

Interactive-Independent Dimension Design Clusters (Greene, 2007)	• Component Mixed Methods Designs:
	  ○ Convergence
	  ○ Extension
	• Integrated Mixed Methods Designs:
	  ○ Iteration
	  ○ Blending
	  ○ Nesting or Embedding
	  ○ Mixing for Reasons of Substance or Values
		• Timing: concurrent or variable
		• Mixing: at results' interpretation
		• Priority: equal or variable
		
		• Timing: concurrent or sequential or variable
		• Mixing: across all stages in a study process
		• Priority: equal or unequal
			This typology:
			• is based on the principles and the purpose of implementation of quantitative and qualitative methods and the weight they carry in the study.
			• is provided by an author writing in the context of evaluation and social sciences.

Five Families of Mixed Methods Designs (Teddlie & Tashakkori, 2009)	• Parallel Mixed Designs • Sequential Mixed Designs	• Timing: concurrent • Mixing: at results' interpretation • Timing: sequential • Mixing: at connecting study phases	This typology: • is based on how quantitative and qualitative methods are mixed within a study. • does not address priority of quantitative and qualitative methods within a study.

	• Conversion Mixed Designs	• Timing: concurrent • Mixing: when transforming one type of data (e.g., qualitative) into an alternative type (e.g., quantitative)	• is provided by the authors writing in the context of social and behavioral research.
	• Multilevel Mixed Designs	• Timing: concurrent or sequential • Mixing: across multiple data levels in a study process	
	• Fully Integrated Mixed Designs	• Timing: concurrent or sequential • Mixing: across all stages in a study process	

Mixed Method Design Typology (Morse & Niehaus, 2009)	• Qualitatively Driven Mixed Method Designs
	  o Qualitatively Driven Simultaneous Designs
	  o Qualitatively Driven Sequential Designs
		• Timing: concurrent or sequential
		• Mixing: at results' interpretation or at connecting two study phases
		• Priority: qualitative
			This typology:
			• is based on the weight and role (core and supplementary) the quantitative and qualitative components play in a study process.
			• is provided by the authors writing in the context of nursing.

	• Quantitatively Driven Mixed Method Designs
	  o Quantitatively Driven Simultaneous Designs
	  o Quantitatively Driven Sequential Designs
		• Timing: concurrent or sequential
		• Mixing: at results' interpretation or at connecting two study phases
		• Priority: quantitative	

	• Complex Mixed and Multiple Method Designs
	  o Qualitatively Driven Designs
	  o Quantitatively Driven Designs
		• Timing: concurrent or sequential
		• Mixing: at connecting multiple study phases
		• Priority: qualitative or quantitative	

(Continued)

Table 5.1 (Continued)

Typologies (Authors)	Mixed Methods Designs	Typical Design Characteristics	Comments
Prototypes of Mixed Methods Designs (Creswell & Plano Clark, 2011)	• Convergent Parallel Mixed Methods Design	• Timing: concurrent • Mixing: at results' interpretation • Priority: equal	This typology: • is based on four methodological decisions: level of interaction, timing, mixing, and priority. • is provided by the authors writing in the context of education and the health sciences.
	• Explanatory Sequential Mixed Methods Design	• Timing: sequential; quantitative first • Mixing: at connecting two study phases • Priority: quantitative	
	• Exploratory Sequential Mixed Methods Design	• Timing: sequential; qualitative first • Mixing: at connecting two study phases • Priority: qualitative	
	• Embedded Mixed Methods Design	• Timing: concurrent or sequential • Mixing: included within a traditional quantitative or qualitative research design • Priority: unequal	
	• Transformative Mixed Methods Design	• Timing: concurrent and sequential • Mixing: at multiple levels as shaped by a theoretical framework • Priority: variable	

	Multiphase Mixed Methods Design		
	• Preliminary Qualitative Input Designs • Preliminary Quantitative Input Designs • Qualitative Follow-Up Designs • Quantitative Follow-Up Designs • Multipart Sequential Designs	• Timing: concurrent and sequential • Mixing: at multiple phases within an overall program-objective framework • Priority: variable	This typology: • is based on the principles of sequencing and prioritizing of quantitative and qualitative methods. • is provided by an author writing in the context of sociology and the health sciences.
Sequential Priorities Model of Mixed Methods Designs (Morgan, 2014)	• Preliminary Qualitative Input Designs	• Timing: sequential; qualitative first • Mixing: at connecting two study phases • Priority: quantitative	
	• Preliminary Quantitative Input Designs	• Timing: sequential; quantitative first • Mixing: at connecting two study phases • Priority: qualitative	
	• Qualitative Follow-Up Designs	• Timing: sequential; quantitative first • Mixing: at connecting two study phases • Priority: quantitative	
	• Quantitative Follow-Up Designs	• Timing: sequential; qualitative first • Mixing: at connecting two study phases • Priority: qualitative	
	• Multipart Sequential Designs	• Timing: sequential; quantitative or qualitative first • Mixing: at connecting multiple study phases • Priority: variable	

A *dynamic approach* to designing a mixed methods study emphasizes the interrelationship of all design components during a study process. For example, Maxwell and Loomis (2003) discussed an interactive, system-based approach to designing a mixed methods study that emphasizes the central role of research questions in a dynamic interaction with all study research components including the conceptual framework, research purpose, methods, and validity considerations. A dynamic approach also provides a more comprehensive approach to designing a mixed methods study in that it tends to be more inclusive of the different epistemological perspectives and skills that researchers and other stakeholders contribute to the study design process. For example, Hall and Howard (2008) advanced a synergistic approach where the design of a mixed methods study underscores the added value of each quantitative and qualitative research method and the multiplied effect of such methodological synergy for a mixed methods study. Similarly, Nastasi, Hitchcock, and Brown (2010) suggested a synergistic partnership-based fully integrated mixed methods research framework for a study design that combined Hall and Howard's (2008) approach with professional collaborative and stakeholder participatory approaches. These dynamic approaches to mixed methods designs emphasize the complexity and interrelationship found among the decisions needed when planning a mixed methods design in contrast to a typology-based approach that emphasizes using prototypical models as guides for design decisions. If you are new to mixed methods research, we suggest you start with a typology-based approach to inform your study design choice based on their purposes and methodological characteristics.

Notation System and Procedural Diagrams

Whichever design approach is used, the resulting mixed methods designs are complex to describe. In response to this complexity, another perspective that has been advanced in the mixed methods literature is related to an increased tendency to use procedural diagrams to effectively communicate mixed methods study designs to readers and grant reviewers. A **procedural diagram** depicts the flow of the research activities in a mixed methods study. It is like a flow chart showing the quantitative and qualitative components and their stages in the study process, the research procedures within each stage, and the outcomes of each stage. Importantly, during a study design, a procedural diagram allows researchers to model the connecting and other integrating points of the quantitative and qualitative study components and plan respective methods' integration procedures. Unfortunately, not all published mixed methods studies include a procedural diagram, which is likely influenced by journal restrictions or researchers' limited training in mixed methods research. In Table 5.2, we included the basic notation symbols used in most procedural diagrams along with their explanations. Many mixed methods texts offer additional symbols, but they vary across the scholars and go beyond the basic designs. These basic notations will assist you in interpreting procedural diagrams found in the literature as well as developing your own procedural diagrams.

Knowing the major perspectives on mixed methods designs will help you better understand different approaches used to conceptualize and design a mixed methods study. It also sets the stage for understanding the underlying

Table 5.2   Notation System for Mixed Methods Procedural Diagrams

Notation	Example	Explanation
Quan, Qual	Quan component Qual component	Capitalized shorthand indicates either a quantitative or qualitative component of a mixed methods study, with no indication of the relative priority.
QUAN, QUAL	QUAN priority QUAL priority	Uppercase letters indicate higher priority of either quantitative or qualitative method in a study.
quan, qual	quan lesser priority qual lesser priority	Lowercase letters indicate lesser priority of either quantitative or qualitative method in a study.
+	QUAN + QUAL	A plus sign indicates that quantitative and qualitative strands are implemented concurrently in a study.
→	QUAN → qual qual → QUAN	An arrow indicates that quantitative and qualitative strands are implemented sequentially in a study.

SOURCE: Based on Morse (1991, 2003).

logics for mixed methods designs that inform the research process in most mixed methods studies. In the following section, we discuss the basic mixed methods design logics, describe the methodological characteristics of three basic mixed methods designs, explain the advantages and challenges of their implementation, and illustrate their application using published mixed methods studies in different disciplines.

BASIC DESIGNS FOR MIXED METHODS RESEARCH

Despite the number and complexity of existing mixed methods design typologies, most mixed methods designs can be described using three basic design logics that we present in Figure 5.2.

Figure 5.2   Three Basic Mixed Methods Design Logics

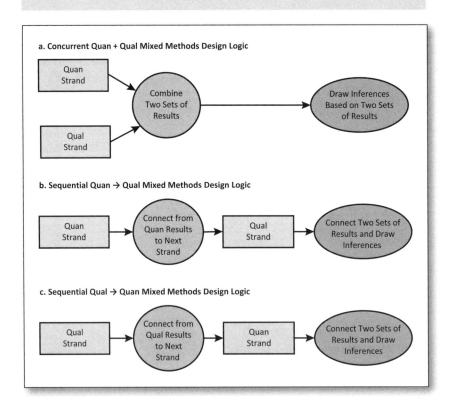

These **mixed methods design logics** encompass a set of essential decisions that researchers have to make when designing a mixed methods research process used in a study. These decisions relate to the timing, integration, and priority of the quantitative and qualitative methods as discussed in Chapter 2. Therefore, mixed methods designs can be viewed as models of the different logics by which quantitative and qualitative methods can be mixed, concurrently or sequentially, to address specific research purposes in a sound, rigorous way.

Each mixed methods design model consists of two strands: a quantitative strand and a qualitative strand. A **strand** is a component of a mixed methods study that encompasses the basic process of conducting quantitative or qualitative research: posing a question, collecting and analyzing data, and interpreting results (Teddlie & Tashakkori, 2009). For example, a quantitative strand of the study is guided by quantitative research questions; it involves gathering numeric data that are analyzed using statistical methods and produce quantitative results. Similarly, a qualitative strand is informed by qualitative research questions and involves collecting qualitative data that are analyzed using inductive thematic approaches to yield qualitative findings.

As shown in Figure 5.2a, the concurrent Quan + Qual design logic implies concurrent timing of the quantitative and qualitative strands. Researchers combine the results from the two strands to draw inferences in response to the posed research questions. The sequential Quan → Qual and Qual → Quan design logics employ sequential timing of the quantitative and qualitative study strands. As depicted in Figures 5.2b and 5.2c, one strand has to be completed before the next strand begins. The order of the strands differs in the two sequential design logics. Researchers connect the two strands when they use the results of one strand to inform the next strand. The two sets of results are also connected at the conclusion of the study to develop inferences to answer the study's research questions.

Using these mixed methods design logics we describe three basic mixed methods designs:

- Concurrent Quan + Qual Design
- Sequential Quan → Qual Design
- Sequential Qual → Quan Design

Concurrent Quan + Qual Design

The **concurrent Quan + Qual design** is a mixed methods design in which researchers implement quantitative and qualitative strands concurrently or independent from each other with the purpose of comparing or merging quantitative and qualitative results to produce more complete and validated conclusions (see Figure 5.2a). The priority is typically given to both methods (QUAN + QUAL), because each method addresses related aspects of the same mixed methods research question in a complementary way. The integration of the quantitative and qualitative methods occurs after the analysis of the data in both study strands is completed and the quantitative and qualitative results are compared or synthesized to find corroborating evidence and to produce a more complete understanding of the research problem. Likewise, researchers can merge data during the analysis stage by way of quantitizing qualitative text data by assigning numeric scores to qualitative codes and themes or by way of qualitizing quantitative numeric data by creating narrative categories based on the distribution of scores. The merged data set is then analyzed using respective quantitative or qualitative methods to produce more substantiated study results.

An advantage of the concurrent Quan + Qual design is that it can produce well-validated and substantiated findings, because concurrent strand implementation allows for obtaining "different but complementary data on the same topic" (Morse, 1991, p. 122). Additionally, researchers can collect and analyze both quantitative and qualitative data within a short period of time, thus saving time and the associated cost for conducting the study (Creswell & Plano Clark, 2011; Morse & Niehaus, 2009). However, this design may be challenging for a solo researcher because of the need to concurrently implement quantitative and qualitative study strands that often require different sets of research skills (Creswell & Plano Clark, 2011; Teddlie & Tashakkori, 2009).

Kawamura, Ivankova, Kohler, and Perumean-Chaney (2009) used the concurrent Quan + Qual design to develop a model that explains how the parasocial interaction between the listeners and the characters in the entertainment–education radio drama BODYLOVE impacts individuals' self-efficacy and practices pertaining to physical exercise. To better communicate the flow of the research activities in their study, Kawamura and colleagues presented the procedural diagram depicted in Figure 5.3. In the quantitative study strand, they tested a hypothesized model via path analysis using the survey data from 105 BODYLOVE program listeners to examine the effect of parasocial interaction on self-efficacy and physical activity practice. During the qualitative strand, they used a grounded theory approach to analyze the interview data from 18 active listeners to understand the role parasocial interaction plays in developing self-efficacy for physical activity. They equally emphasized quantitative (survey) and qualitative (interview) data because both data sets were similarly important in addressing the research purpose. In the final stage, the two models that the researchers developed in the quantitative (path analysis) and qualitative (grounded theory) study strands were combined using "triangulation and complementarity in the integration process" to create a composite model explaining the program's influence on listeners' physical activity practice (p. 88).

Figure 5.3   A Procedural Diagram of Research Activities in
Kawamura et al.'s (2009) Concurrent Quan + Qual Study

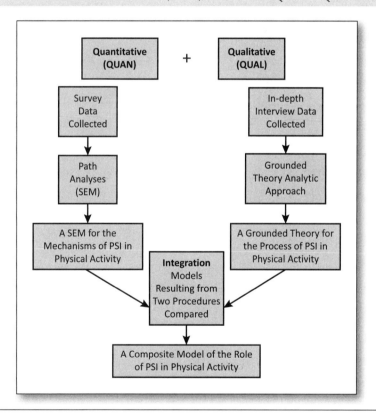

SOURCE: Kawamura, Y., Ivankova, N., Kohler, C., & Perumean-Chaney, S. (2009). Utilizing mixed methods to assess parasocial interaction of one entertainment–education program audience. *International Journal of Multiple Research Approaches, 3*(1), 88–104. doi:10.5172/mra.455.3.1.88. Reprinted by permission of Taylor & Francis Ltd.

NOTE: SEM = structural equation modeling; PSI = parasocial interaction.

Sequential Quan → Qual Design

The **sequential Quan → Qual design** is a mixed methods design in which researchers implement quantitative and qualitative strands in sequence with the purpose of using follow-up qualitative data to elaborate, explain, or confirm the initial quantitative results (see Figure 5.2b). The priority may be given to the quantitative (QUAN → qual) or qualitative (quan → QUAL) study strands depending on the study focus. The mixing of the quantitative and qualitative methods occurs at two points: (1) when the two study strands are connected after the completion of the quantitative strand and beginning of the qualitative strand and (2) when the results from both study strands are interpreted together. For example, researchers can use the results from the quantitative survey in the first strand to identify individuals for follow-up qualitative interviews in the second strand and then interpret the two sets of results together so that the qualitative findings can provide better understanding of the initial quantitative results.

An advantage of the sequential Quan → Qual design is that the chrono-logical sequence of the quantitative and qualitative strands makes it more straightforward and easy to implement by one researcher (Creswell & Plano Clark, 2011; Ivankova, Creswell, & Stick, 2006; Morgan, 2014; Morse & Niehaus, 2009). This design also provides an opportunity for the exploration of the initial quantitative results in more detail, especially when unexpected results arise from a quantitative strand (Morse, 1991). The limitations of this design are related to the length of time of the study implementation and the challenge of recontacting participants in the second follow-up strand.

Mayoh, Bond, and Todres (2012) employed the sequential Quan → Qual design to study the online health information (OHI) seeking experiences of older adults with chronic health conditions. They presented the study's design in the procedural diagram that we depicted in Figure 5.4. They adopted a sequential approach to first identify quantitative patterns of the OHI-seeking experiences and then gain deeper understanding using qualitative methods. The aim of the first, quantitative strand (Phase 1) was to examine the prevalence, characteristics, and outcomes of OHI seeking by surveying 100 older adults attending support groups for chronic health conditions in the United Kingdom. Researchers included both closed- and open-ended questions in the survey instrument, which they indicated in their diagram with the shorthand "quanqual questionnaire." The aim of the subsequent qualitative strand (Phase 2) was "to obtain in-depth qualitative descriptions of the OHI-seeking experiences for older adults, with reference to six appropriate and specific experiences that were outlined as relevant by Phase I" (p. 27). To achieve this aim, Mayoh and colleagues interviewed six individuals about six different types of OHI-seeking experiences and analyzed the qualitative data using a phenomenological approach. The authors did not discuss which method they prioritized in the study, but it seems they emphasized the quantitative strand based on the amount of data collected to identify six different prototypes of OHI-seeking/sharing experiences. They integrated the two sets of results by using qualitative themes to support and extend the statistical results, thus providing a more clear understanding of the complex phenomenon of OHI-seeking.

Sequential Qual → Quan Design

The **sequential Qual → Quan design** is a mixed methods design in which researchers implement qualitative and quantitative strands in sequence with the purpose of using follow-up quantitative data to generalize, test, or

Figure 5.4   A Procedural Diagram of Research Activities in Mayoh et al.'s (2012) Sequential Quan → Qual Study

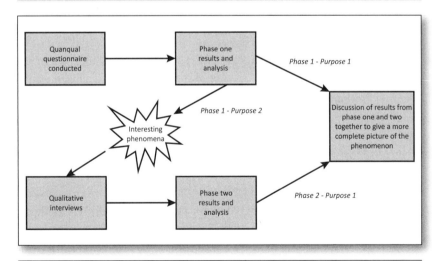

SOURCE: Mayoh, J., Bond, C. S, & Todres, L. (2012). An innovative mixed methods approach to studying the online health information seeking experiences of adults with chronic health conditions. *Journal of Mixed Methods Research, 6*(1), 21–33. Reprinted with permission.

confirm initial qualitative results (see Figure 5.2c). Priority can be given to either the qualitative (QUAL → quan) or quantitative (qual → QUAN) study strand in this design. The mixing of the methods occurs chronologically at the completion of the first, qualitative strand and beginning of the second, quantitative strand and also when the results from both study strands are interpreted together. For example, researchers can use the results from qualitative interviews to inform the development and administration of a new survey instrument and then interpret the two sets of results together so that the quantitative results can verify, confirm, or generalize the initial exploratory qualitative findings.

Likewise, an advantage of the sequential Qual → Quan design is that due to the chronological sequence of the qualitative and quantitative strands, the study unfolds in a more predictable manner and makes it easy for one researcher to implement (Teddlie & Tashakkori, 2009). This design is specifically useful in situations when researchers want to explore the phenomenon in depth with a few individuals but also want to expand these findings to a larger population. The sequential nature of this design also may require lengthy time and more resources to collect and analyze both sets of data. Additionally, developing a measurement instrument is a complex process that requires adherence to special psychometric procedures.

Moubarac, Cargo, Receveur, and Daniel (2012) used the sequential Qual → Quan design to describe the situational contexts associated with the consumption of sweetened products in a Catholic Middle Eastern Canadian community. They presented a detailed procedural diagram of the study's activities including steps, procedures, and products that we depicted in Figure 5.5. Moubarac and colleagues adopted this design to identify themes describing the situational contexts of sweetened product consumption to inform the development of the quantitative survey instrument. They considered the strength of this design in using quantitative methods to complement qualitative methods so that to identify and describe the studied phenomenon "where findings from the quantitative data were compared with qualitative results" (p. e44738). The authors did not discuss the priority of the methods, but based on the purpose of this design and the role of the qualitative data in informing the development of the new instrument to measure sweetened product consumption, we believe the authors gave more emphasis to the qualitative method. In the first, qualitative strand, they conducted semi-structured interviews with 42 community residents and used the themes and items from

Figure 5.5   A Procedural Diagram of Research Activities in
Moubarac et al.'s (2012) Sequential Qual → Quan Study

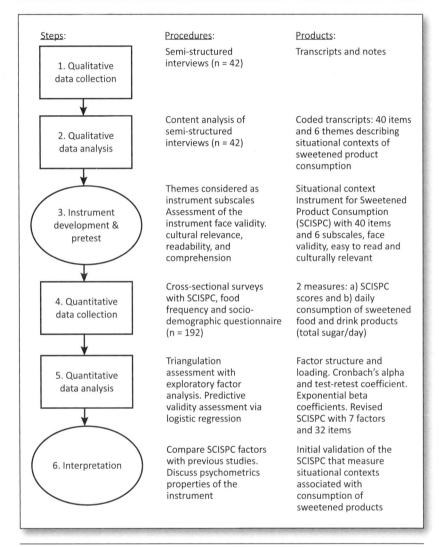

Steps:	Procedures:	Products:
1. Qualitative data collection	Semi-structured interviews (n = 42)	Transcripts and notes
2. Qualitative data analysis	Content analysis of semi-structured interviews (n = 42)	Coded transcripts: 40 items and 6 themes describing situational contexts of sweetened product consumption
3. Instrument development & pretest	Themes considered as instrument subscales Assessment of the instrument face validity. cultural relevance, readability, and comprehension	Situational context Instrument for Sweetened Product Consumption (SCISPC) with 40 items and 6 subscales, face validity, easy to read and culturally relevant
4. Quantitative data collection	Cross-sectional surveys with SCISPC, food frequency and socio-demographic questionnaire (n = 192)	2 measures: a) SCISPC scores and b) daily consumption of sweetened food and drink products (total sugar/day)
5. Quantitative data analysis	Triangulation assessment with exploratory factor analysis. Predictive validity assessment via logistic regression	Factor structure and loading. Cronbach's alpha and test-retest coefficient. Exponential beta coefficients. Revised SCISPC with 7 factors and 32 items
6. Interpretation	Compare SCISPC factors with previous studies. Discuss psychometrics properties of the instrument	Initial validation of the SCISPC that measure situational contexts associated with consumption of sweetened products

SOURCE: Moubarac, J. C., Cargo, M., Receveur, O., & Daniel, M. (2012). Describing the situational contexts of sweetened product consumption in a Middle Eastern Canadian community: Application of a mixed method design. *PLoS ONE* 7(9), e44738. doi:10.1371/journal .pone.0044738. Retrieved from http://journals.plos.org/plosone/article?id=10.1371/journal .pone.0044738.

content analysis as a foundation for developing the instrument subscales and items. In the subsequent quantitative strand, they administered the new instrument to 192 members from the same church communities and conducted its construct validation. At the study conclusion, they discussed the implications for the prevention and management of obesity in the Middle Eastern Canadian community grounded in the two sets of results.

ISSUES AND DEBATES ABOUT THE MIXED METHODS RESEARCH DESIGNS

The three basic designs that we have discussed and illustrated in this chapter provide a simple typology for describing the different logics commonly used in mixed methods research. That said, mixed methods designs remain one of the most debated topics in the mixed methods research literature. Consensus does not exist among scholars about how best to describe and delineate the major mixed methods designs and what criteria should be considered in guiding the choice of the design. With many different perspectives on mixed methods designs that exist in the field, it becomes very difficult for novice researchers both to understand different applications of mixed methods and to make informed decisions about what design to use for their mixed methods studies and how to justify this selection. Here, we introduce some of the issues about mixed methods research designs that continue to be discussed and debated within the field of mixed methods research.

1. Do we need mixed methods design typologies? Although many mixed methods scholars have been involved in developing typologies of mixed methods designs, there are divergent opinions about their purposes and utility. Some scholars see design typologies as useful because they outline the design features common to a group of mixed methods studies and can help researchers make more informed decisions when choosing an approach for designing their study in response to a specific research question (Creswell & Plano Clark, 2011; Greene et al., 1989; Teddlie & Tashakkori, 2009). Another point of view is that no typology can capture all possible variations in designing mixed methods studies because a study design is driven by a unique research problem that requires gathering information to answer the posed research questions within the parameters of this problem

(Greene, 2007; Hall & Howard, 2008; Maxwell & Loomis, 2003). There is a recent tendency toward "the reconceptualization of research designs away from typologies" (Creswell, 2010, p. 59). The argument is that typologies are overemphasized and that researchers should focus on considering and describing the design decisions that they have made to address a specific research purpose (Bazeley, 2009; Guest, 2013). We suggest you weigh the advantages and limitations of a typology-based approach when you consider how to identify your approach to mixed methods designs.

   2. What criteria should be considered in choosing a mixed methods design? There is consensus among mixed methods scholars that mixed methods designs are unique and have their own methodological dimensions. However, there are different opinions with regard to what decisions researchers should make when conceptualizing a study design (Tashakkori, 2009). For example, not all scholars agree that priority of the quantitative or qualitative approach should be an important design consideration. One view is that the relative importance or status of the quantitative and qualitative study strands within the design is predetermined by the research purpose (Creswell & Plano Clark, 2011; Greene, 2007; Leech & Onwuegbuzie, 2009; Morgan, 2014). An alternative view suggests that the priority of the method is often flexible and cannot be determined before the study is completed (Teddlie & Tashakkori, 2009). Similarly, scholars disagree whether the purposes of quantitative and qualitative methods' integration suggested by Greene and colleagues (1989) should be a design feature since these are "the functions of the research study" and cannot be defined a priori (Teddlie & Tashakkori, 2009, p. 140). Morse and Niehaus (2009) provided a different consideration when they advanced the idea of a study's theoretical drive that informs the type of the mixed methods design used. We suggest you carefully consider the methodological dimensions of mixed methods designs that we described in this chapter when you decide what design characteristics to emphasize in your mixed methods research practice.

   3. Should there be *one* name for the same mixed methods research design? Scholars writing about mixed methods research have developed numerous typologies of mixed methods designs that added to the complexity of the field. As we showed with five prominent typologies included in Table 5.1, different typologies often include similar designs that are labeled differently. The authors of the typologies use different methodological considerations for naming the designs, such as timing, mixing, and the role quantitative and qualitative methods play in the study. Additionally, the same designs have been reconceptualized over the years and continue to be referred to by different names in the literature; for example, concurrent, simultaneous, and triangulation designs (Teddlie & Tashakkori, 2010). We suggest you pay attention to the design names and the methodological characteristics that the authors emphasize in naming their designs when you read, review, or design mixed methods research.

These three questions highlight important issues and debates related to designs for mixed methods research. They also indicate the importance for researchers to clearly define their approach to mixed methods designs and the criteria they use in selecting an appropriate design to address the study's research questions. While these debates add to the controversies in the mixed methods field and make it more difficult for researchers to navigate, they are viewed as healthy signs of the field development. As Tashakkori (2009) pointed out, "Creating bridges between various conceptualizations of integrated research designs might be more difficult, but it is possible" (p. 289).

APPLYING THE MIXED METHODS RESEARCH DESIGNS IN RESEARCH PRACTICE

As we have shown, mixed methods designs have a direct impact on how researchers approach the mixed methods research process. Choosing and/or developing an appropriate design is a key methodological consideration in a mixed methods study because it has implications for how researchers implement the quantitative and qualitative strands and how they generate inferences from the integrated quantitative and qualitative results. Taking into account the complexity of existing mixed methods design typologies and a plethora of views on the criteria for choosing a mixed methods design, it is important for you to be able to recognize and articulate the basic designs and their underlying logic. Understanding the design logic and decisions involved in the process of a study design will help you read about, plan, conduct, report, and evaluate mixed methods studies. Box 5.1 includes our advice for applying the concepts of this chapter to your mixed methods research practice.

Box 5.1

Advice for Applying the Mixed Methods Research Designs in Research Practice

Advice for Reading/Reviewing Mixed Methods Studies and Methodological Discussions

- Keep in mind that the basic mixed methods designs serve as models of the logic by which quantitative and qualitative methods can be mixed—concurrently or sequentially—to address specific research purposes.
- When reading about and reviewing applications of basic mixed methods designs, consider the major perspectives about designs for mixed methods research and how they might influence how researchers approached designing mixed methods studies.
- Note how the authors defined the employed mixed methods design and how they used the mixed methods literature to justify their approach.
- Assess if the authors clearly articulated the purpose of the mixed methods design and the reasons for using it.
- Assess how the authors described the mixed methods design, including the design logic and the timing, integration, and priority of the quantitative and qualitative study strands.
- Note if the authors provided the procedural diagram of the research activities in the study.
- Assess how the authors drew inferences using the design logic for integrating quantitative and qualitative methods to address the study's research questions.

Advice for Proposing/Reporting/Discussing Mixed Methods Research

- Clearly articulate the mixed methods design and the reasons for using it in your study, citing relevant mixed methods literature.
- Describe the chosen mixed methods design, including the design logic and the timing, integration, and priority of the quantitative and qualitative study strands.

(Continued)

(Continued)

- Include a procedural diagram of the research activities in the study to effectively communicate the logical flow of the procedures to the readers.
- Explain how each study strand is implemented including sampling, data collection, and analysis, using sound quantitative and qualitative research methods.
- Discuss how you draw inferences using the design logic for integrating quantitative and qualitative methods to address the study's research questions.

When reading and reviewing the literature about mixed methods research, it is essential to pay particular attention to how researchers approach designing their studies. It is useful to remember that most mixed methods studies make use of the basic mixed methods designs that provide the underlying logic for integrating the quantitative and qualitative methods during a study process. However, researchers may adopt different perspectives on mixed methods designs that might influence how they approach designing their mixed methods studies. So it is important to note how the authors defined the employed mixed methods design and how they used the mixed methods literature to justify their approach. No matter what approach to designing a mixed methods study—typology-based or dynamic—the authors used to inform their study design, it is important to assess how they described the study's design, including the design logic and the timing, integration, and priority of the quantitative and qualitative study strands. It is equally important to note how the authors drew final inferences to answer the study's research questions and whether the inferences result from the integration of the quantitative and qualitative methods in the study. Finally, pay attention if the authors provided a procedural diagram to effectively communicate the research activities in the study.

It is equally important to identify your approach to mixed methods designs when you design and report your own mixed methods research study. Readers who will review and evaluate your study will benefit if you clearly articulate the mixed methods design and the reasons for using it, citing supporting mixed methods literature. You are expected to describe the chosen mixed methods design in detail, including the design logic and the timing, integration, and priority of the quantitative and qualitative study strands. It is recommended that you include a procedural diagram of the research activities in the study to effectively communicate the logical flow of the procedures to the readers. Explain how each study strand is implemented with the focus on sampling, data collection, and analysis, using sound quantitative and qualitative research methods. Describe how you draw inferences, using the design logic for integrating quantitative and qualitative methods to address the posed research questions. By fully explaining your mixed methods research design to the readers they will be in a better position to understand and evaluate your mixed methods study.

CONCLUDING COMMENTS

We conclude the chapter by offering some final summary comments organized by the learning objectives stated at the beginning of the chapter.

- **Understand different perspectives about designs for mixed methods research.** The major views on mixed methods designs include distinguishing between truly mixed and quasi-mixed designs and fixed and emergent designs. Additionally, researchers can choose from typology-based and dynamic approaches to designing mixed methods studies. Scholars have introduced notations and procedural diagrams to facilitate the description of mixed methods designs.
- **Describe three basic mixed methods designs and their underlying logic.** Mixed methods designs are models of the logic by which quantitative and qualitative methods can be mixed—concurrently or sequentially—to address specific research purposes. Most mixed methods studies make use of the three basic mixed methods designs: concurrent Quan + Qual, sequential Quan → Qual, and sequential Qual → Quan.
- **Understand how the basic mixed methods designs are applied in research practice**. When applying mixed methods designs, researchers should consider the designs' logic; characteristics, such as timing, integration, and priority; and advantages and challenges of implementation. Procedural diagrams that depict the flow of the research activities in a study can help researchers effectively communicate their mixed methods designs.

APPLICATION QUESTIONS

1. Reflect on the major perspectives about designs for mixed methods research discussed in this chapter including truly vs. quasi-mixed designs, fixed vs. emergent designs, and typology-based vs. dynamic approaches to design. Discuss how each of these perspectives may shape your approach to designing a mixed methods study. Explain which approach appeals to you most and why.

2. Locate a mixed methods published study in your discipline or area of interest. Carefully read the study reflecting on how the study was designed and implemented. For this study, do the following:

   a. Identify the type of basic mixed methods design used.

   b. Consider how the authors described the choice of the design and what mixed methods literature they cited to support their choice.

   c. Discuss the design logic and how timing, integration, and priority of the quantitative and qualitative study strands were addressed in the study.

   d. Reflect on how well the chosen mixed methods design helped address the study's research purpose and questions.

   e. Consider if the authors provided a procedural diagram of their design. Discuss how well the diagram captures the mixed methods procedures in the study.

   f. Using the notation system introduced in this chapter, draw your own procedural diagram for the study.

3. Choose one issue from the ongoing issues and debates about mixed methods research designs: the need for design typologies, the best way to choose a design, or the names for designs. State why you selected that issue, and discuss your reactions to it in terms of how this issue might affect the way you read about, plan, conduct, report, and evaluate mixed methods studies.

KEY RESOURCES

To learn more about mixed methods research designs, we suggest you start with the following resources:

1. **Teddlie, C., & Tashakkori, A. (2009). Mixed methods research designs. In** *Foundations of mixed methods research: Integrating quantitative and qualitative approaches in the social and behavioral sciences* **(pp. 137–167). Thousand Oaks, CA: Sage.**

   - In this chapter, Teddlie and Tashakkori introduced five major types of mixed methods designs, described other typologies of mixed methods designs, and advanced the seven-step process for selecting a mixed methods design.

2. **Creswell, J. W., & Plano Clark, V. L. (2011). Choosing a mixed methods design. In** *Designing and conducting mixed methods research* **(2nd ed., pp. 53–68). Thousand Oaks, CA: Sage.**

   - In this chapter, Creswell and Plano Clark discussed the principles of designing a mixed methods study, introduced the basic types of mixed methods designs, and described the decisions in choosing a mixed methods design.

3. **Morse, J. M., & Niehaus, L. (2009). The nuts and bolts of mixed method design. In** *Mixed method design: Principles and procedures* **(pp. 23–37)*. Walnut Creek, CA: Left Coast Press.**

   - In this chapter, Morse and Niehaus introduced basic mixed method designs, described their main components, and discussed some design pitfalls that researchers should be aware of.

*4. **Guest, G. (2013). Describing mixed methods research: An alternative to typologies.** *Journal of Mixed Methods Research, 7*(2), **141–151.**

   - In this article, Guest addressed the debate about the existence of and the need for mixed methods design typologies. The author suggested an alternative way of describing mixed methods studies using only two dimensions—the timing and the purpose of data integration.

∗ The key resource is available at the following website: http://study.sagepub.com/planoclark.

✠ SIX ✠

HOW TO EXPAND THE USE OF MIXED METHODS RESEARCH?

INTERSECTING MIXED METHODS WITH OTHER APPROACHES

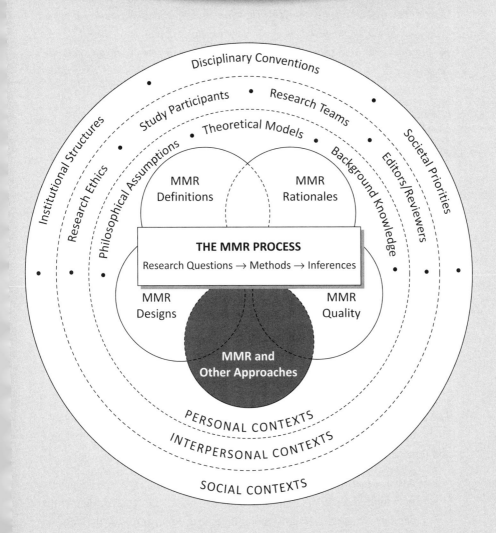

*N*ow that you have been introduced to the three basic mixed methods designs, you can recognize and describe the logic used to integrate the quantitative and qualitative methods in most mixed methods studies. There are situations, however, where researchers expand the use of mixed methods beyond the basic designs by intersecting mixed methods research with other research designs, methodological approaches, and theoretical frameworks. We consider these hybrid approaches to be advanced applications of mixed methods designs because they add additional considerations to the use of mixed methods. Advanced applications of mixed methods designs provide researchers with a broad array of methodological possibilities for their studies and are discussed across extensive writings in the field. Therefore, to help you understand and navigate the full range of mixed methods designs, this chapter describes different perspectives for and examples of how researchers intersect mixed methods research with other approaches and frameworks.

LEARNING OBJECTIVES

This chapter aims to provide you with an understanding of how mixed methods research can intersect with other approaches and frameworks so you are able to do the following:

- Describe advanced applications of mixed methods designs.
- Understand different perspectives about the ways in which mixed methods research can intersect with other research designs, methodological approaches, and theoretical frameworks.
- Consider how several different advanced applications of mixed methods designs are used in research practice.

CHAPTER 6 KEY CONCEPTS

The following key concepts will help you navigate through the main considerations related to intersecting mixed methods research with other approaches and frameworks as they are introduced in this chapter:

- **Advanced applications of mixed methods designs:** Hybrid approaches in which researchers intersect a basic mixed methods design with another research design, methodological approach, or theoretical framework.

- **Research design:** A formal and defined set of research procedures for collecting, analyzing, and interpreting data to address a specific type of study purpose.
- **Methodological approach:** An established set of general perspectives and procedures that guide the design and conduct of research.
- **Theoretical framework:** An abstract and formalized set of assumptions and stances about the social world used to guide the design and conduct of research.
- **Intersecting:** Intentionally embedding or joining two or more research designs, methodological approaches, and/or theoretical frameworks within a study's mixed methods research design.
- **Embedding (or nesting):** Incorporating a secondary method (quantitative or qualitative) within a research design traditionally associated with the other approach (qualitative or quantitative).
- **Mixed methods experiment:** A research design in which researchers embed qualitative methods within a quantitative experimental design to enhance the application of the experiment for testing the effects of an intervention.
- **Mixed methods case study:** A research design in which researchers embed quantitative methods within a qualitative case study design to enhance the application of the case study for describing and interpreting a case.
- **Mixed methods evaluation:** A research approach in which researchers integrate quantitative and qualitative methods within an evaluation methodological approach to enhance the application of this approach for addressing the evaluation goals.
- **Mixed methods action research:** A research approach in which researchers integrate quantitative and qualitative methods within an action research methodological approach to enhance the application of action research for solving the practical problem of interest.
- **Transformative mixed methods research:** A research approach in which researchers integrate quantitative and qualitative methods within a social justice theoretical framework to enhance the application of research for addressing a social justice agenda.

THE ROLE OF ADVANCED APPLICATIONS OF DESIGNS IN THE FIELD OF MIXED METHODS RESEARCH

As introduced in Chapter 5, most mixed methods studies make use of three basic mixed methods designs. These basic designs provide the underlying logic for integrating the quantitative and qualitative strands of a study concurrently or sequentially. In some situations, researchers choose to conduct more complex mixed methods designs that consist of multiple strands and combine two or more basic sequential and concurrent designs. Although many research questions can be adequately addressed by using one or more basic mixed methods designs, there are other situations where researchers choose to use advanced applications of mixed methods designs. We define *advanced applications of mixed methods designs* as hybrid approaches in which researchers intersect a basic mixed methods design with another research design, methodological approach, or theoretical framework (Creswell, 2015; Creswell & Plano Clark, 2011). Although there are many possible meanings for several of these terms, the following definitions guide our use of these terms in this chapter. A **research design** is a formal and defined set of procedures for collecting, analyzing, and interpreting data to address a specific type of research purpose. Examples of research designs include quantitative experiments and qualitative case studies. A **methodological approach** is an established set of general perspectives and procedures that guide the design and conduct of research. Examples of methodological approaches include action research, social network analysis, and evaluation research. A **theoretical framework** is an abstract and formalized set of assumptions and stances about the social world used to guide the design and conduct of research. Examples of theoretical frameworks (sometimes referred to as grand theories) include feminism, critical race theory, and positive psychology.

When researchers use a hybrid design, they add a level of complexity to their use of mixed methods by intentionally **intersecting** (embedding or joining) a mixed methods design with another research design, methodological approach, or theoretical framework. For example, researchers might intersect their use of mixed methods with a quantitative experiment design, with a qualitative case study design, with an evaluation approach, with an action research approach, or with a feminist theoretical framework. Each of these approaches and frameworks is associated with its own set of assumptions and logics for conducting research. Therefore, mixed methods designs that intersect with approaches such as these are considered "advanced" applications because researchers need to consider and navigate additional assumptions and logics in their use of mixed methods and not because these designs necessarily use more sophisticated methods and procedures.

By intersecting mixed methods with other approaches and frameworks, scholars also bring a mixed methods way of thinking to another well-established approach (such as thinking about social network analysis from a mixed methods perspective or using mixed methods to inform the stages in the action research cycle) in addition to increasing the nuances associated with the application of mixed methods research. Because of the multitude of possibilities that exist for intersecting mixed methods with other approaches, hybrid approaches are becoming of increasing interest and encouraging expanding growth in the field of mixed methods as they bring many new scholars from different disciplines to the field (Creswell, 2010). As illustrated in Figure 6.1, the intersection of mixed methods with other approaches provides many additional possible approaches for mixed methods research practice—each of which directly influences the mixed methods research process used in a study. Therefore, to understand the full range of mixed methods designs possible, you need to recognize and understand the use of advanced applications of mixed methods designs in addition to the basic mixed methods designs.

Figure 6.1 The Role of Advanced Applications of Designs in the Practice of Mixed Methods Research

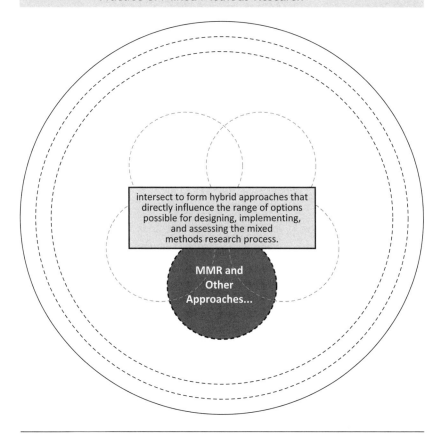

NOTE: MMR = mixed methods research.

MAJOR PERSPECTIVES ABOUT ADVANCED
APPLICATIONS OF DESIGNS FOR MIXED METHODS RESEARCH

Due to the potential value and possible variations of advanced applications of mixed methods designs, scholars have considered a diverse range of definitions, issues, and applications of these approaches within the field of mixed methods research. Although the literature about advanced applications of designs is extensive, there is actually little consensus within this literature about how to label or describe designs that intersect mixed methods research with other approaches. As we have examined this expanding literature, we have found it useful to conceptualize the ongoing discussions in terms of three overarching perspectives about what it means to intersect other approaches with mixed methods research. Although there is frequently some overlap among the three perspectives, they effectively summarize the different ways that scholars discuss and use advanced applications of mixed methods designs. These perspectives, which are illustrated in Figure 6.2 and discussed in the following sections, are as follows:

- Embedding a secondary method within a primary quantitative or qualitative research design
- Mixing methods within a methodological approach
- Mixing methods within a theoretical framework

Embedding a Secondary Method Within
a Primary Quantitative or Qualitative Research Design

One of the earliest perspectives articulated in the literature for how mixed methods might intersect with another approach is the concept of embedding. **Embedding** (or **nesting**) refers to a mixed methods approach in which a researcher incorporates a secondary method (quantitative or qualitative) within a research design traditionally associated with the other approach (qualitative or quantitative) (Caracelli & Greene, 1997; Creswell & Plano Clark, 2011; Creswell, Plano Clark, Gutmann, & Hanson, 2003; Greene, 2007; Plano Clark et al., 2013). Caracelli and Greene (1997) first described embedding as a design that features "one methodology located within another, interlocking contrasting inquiry characteristics in a framework of creative tension" (p. 24). In Figure 6.2a, we provide two options for how the embedded mixed methods approach is conceptualized. The left nested ovals depict a qualitative method (e.g., interviews and thematic analysis) located within a

Figure 6.2   Three Perspectives for How Mixed Methods Research Can Intersect With Other Approaches

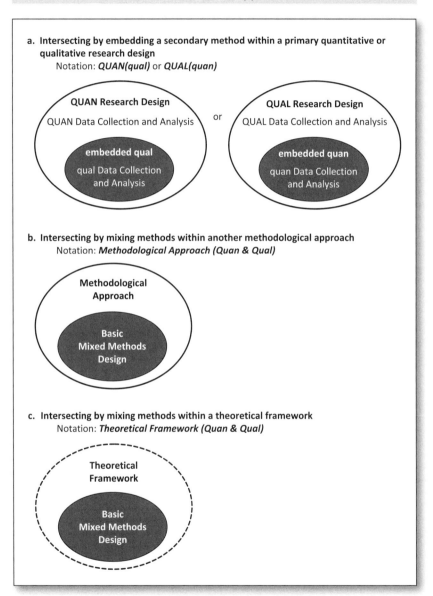

NOTE: Uppercase letters QUAN or QUAL = primary research design and overall study priority; Lowercase letters quan or qual = secondary method with lesser priority; Quan & Qual = any basic mixed methods design (concurrent or sequential timing, equal or unequal priority)

primary quantitative research design (e.g., an experimental or longitudinal panel design). The right nested ovals depict a quantitative method (e.g., survey questionnaires and correlational analysis) located within a primary qualitative research design (e.g., an ethnographic or case study design).

When using an embedded mixed methods approach, researchers clearly design their studies using a traditional quantitative or qualitative research design but then choose to add a secondary method that is complementary, supplementary, and in service to the primary design. As such, embedded designs are noted for having unequal priority where the approach associated with the primary design has priority and the secondary method has a lesser weight. Greene (2007) further explained the relationship between the two methods in an embedded design by noting that the embedded secondary method "follows or adheres to key parameters of the primary method—for example, sampling or designed controls—rather than following the parameters usually associated with this secondary method" (pp. 127–128). That is, the secondary embedded method is designed so that it fits the methodological requirements of the primary research design. On the one hand, if a qualitative method is embedded in a quantitative experimental design, then the use of that qualitative method will follow the experimental design characteristics and will adhere to a high level of control that is required so as not to bias the experiment. For example, Plano Clark and colleagues (2013) described how they embedded qualitative methods within an experiment designed to test the effects of two doses of a psychoeducational intervention for oncology patients with pain. To meet the experiment's requirements and not introduce confounding factors, they only gathered unobtrusive forms of qualitative data by recording the conversations that occurred as part of the intervention, kept the qualitative data collection forms fixed for the entire experiment, and gathered the qualitative data from all participants (despite the very large sample size). On the other hand, if a quantitative method is embedded in a qualitative case study design, then the quantitative sample will likely be very small and purposefully selected because it is limited to those individuals who are part of the case. For example, Evans, Belyea, and Ume (2011) embedded a quantitative measure over time for a sample of only two participants in their multiple case study design to enrich the two case descriptions.

Mixing Methods Within a Methodological Approach

A more recent perspective about intersecting mixed methods with other approaches is the idea of mixing methods within a specific methodological approach (Creswell, 2010, 2015; Ivankova, 2015). In contrast to embedding that focuses on adding a secondary method to a quantitative or a qualitative research design (see Figure 6.2a), this perspective focuses on bringing a mixed methods way of thinking to an existing methodological approach—that is, a researcher implements a basic mixed methods design within a specific methodological approach (see Figure 6.2b). For example, a researcher might mix quantitative and qualitative methods within an evaluation approach or within an action research approach or within a social network analysis approach. When discussing this perspective, Creswell (2010) noted that the overarching methodological approach can be viewed as a "placeholder" (p. 52) for mixing methods, with the integration of quantitative and qualitative strands occurring within that approach. The use of mixed methods is shaped by and adapted to the parameters associated with the overarching method-ological approach as a means for enhancing the ability to address the research purpose.

Building from this perspective, the potential for expanding the designs for mixed methods has been described as "staggering" (Creswell, 2010, p. 52). This expansion is already readily apparent in the literature where we find examples of scholars writing about and researchers using mixed methods within many other methodological approaches. Examples of the wide variety of ways that scholars are mixing methods within other research approaches include the fol-lowing: mixed methods and longitudinal research (Plano Clark et al., 2014; Van Ness, Fried, & Gill, 2011), mixed methods and Q methodology (Newman & Ramlo, 2010), mixed methods and phenomenological research (Mayoh & Onwuegbuzie, 2015), mixed methods and grounded theory research (Johnson, McGowan, & Turner, 2010), mixed methods and action research (Ivankova, 2015; Phillips & Davidson, 2009), mixed methods and evaluation approaches (Bamberger, Rao, & Woolcock, 2010; Nastasi et al., 2007), mixed methods and research syntheses (Harden & Thomas, 2010; Heyvaert, Maes, & Onghena, 2013; Sandelowski, Voils, Leeman, & Crandell, 2012), mixed methods and biographical research (Nilsen & Brannen, 2010), and mixed method and social network analysis (Edwards, 2010). It is true that many of these methodological approaches have always had the potential to combine quantitative and qualita-tive methods. For example, evaluation approaches have often used qualitative methods to perform formative assessments about the implementation of pro-grams combined with quantitative methods to perform summative assessments of the outcomes of programs. However, many such examples from the past may have included both methods, but they did not necessarily integrate the methods as is done in the basic mixed methods designs. In contrast, scholars such as those cited earlier in this paragraph are bringing a mixed methods perspective to these other methodological approaches—that is, these scholars not only use quantitative and qualitative methods within an established methodological approach but also emphasize the integration of those methods within that approach thus enhancing its application.

Mixing Methods Within a Theoretical Framework

A third perspective about intersecting mixed methods with other approaches is the idea of mixing methods within a theoretical framework (Caracelli & Greene, 1997; Creswell & Plano Clark, 2011; Creswell et al., 2003; Mertens, 2003; Mertens, Bledsoe, Sullivan, & Wilson, 2010). This perspective emphasizes a theory-driven (or ideological) orientation to using mixed methods (see Figure 6.2c) in contrast to a methodological approach (see Figures 6.2a and 6.2b). For example, a researcher working from a social justice theoretical framework (such as feminism or critical race theory) whose intent is to uncover and challenge unjust practices may use that framework to directly shape all of the decisions about how mixed methods is designed and implemented. As Caracelli and Greene (1997) described, when researchers use mixed methods within a theoretical framework, they "give primacy to the value-based and action-oriented dimensions of different inquiry traditions" (Caracelli & Greene, 1997, p. 24).

The mixed methods literature includes numerous discussions of the meaning and value of intersecting mixed methods research with different theoretical frameworks. These discussions are most often framed in terms of an overarching social justice theory guiding the researchers' assumptions and research approaches. For example, scholars have discussed how mixed methods research can intersect with and be adapted to feminism (Hesse-Biber, 2010a, 2012; Oakley, 1998), intersectionality theory (Harper, 2011; Maramba & Museus, 2011), and critical viewpoints (Greene, 2012; Onwuegbuzie & Frels, 2013). Less commonly, scholars have also written about the intersection of mixed methods with other types of theoretical frameworks besides those associated with social justice perspectives (e.g., Creswell et al., 2003; Greene, 2007). Examples of such theoretical frameworks include strengths-based theory (Lietz, 2009) and framing theory (Parmelee, Perkins, & Sayre, 2007).

It is important to note that all of these theories (and the many more not listed here) can be used with most any research methodology, including mixed methods. When scholars discuss mixing methods within a theoretical framework, they are choosing to elevate the primacy of the theoretical orientation to the research and its influence on the use of the basic mixed methods designs. The distinction between "mixing methods within a theoretical framework" and "using a theory in a mixed methods research study" is not always easy to determine. The key point here from the perspective of intersecting mixed methods with a theoretical framework is that everything about the study, including the use of mixed methods, is considered and framed from the researchers' stance as articulated by the overarching theoretical framework. Therefore, researchers using this approach will likely make decisions about the application of mixed methods for different reasons than those typically associated with the basic mixed methods designs.

EXAMPLES OF INTERSECTING MIXED METHODS WITH OTHER APPROACHES

As demonstrated by the three perspectives described in the previous section, there are countless ways in which researchers can intersect mixed methods with other approaches and frameworks to form advanced applications of mixed methods designs. The literature describes many of these possibilities, and the list continues to grow and expand. Here, we provide brief introductions to five advanced applications of mixed methods designs that we have found to be more extensively used in research practice and discussed in the literature. We refer to these hybrid approaches as mixed methods experiments, mixed methods case studies, mixed methods evaluation, mixed methods action research, and transformative mixed methods research.

Mixed Methods Experiment

Experiments (including intervention trials and quasi-experiments) are quantitative research designs in which researchers control the conditions experienced by participants, administer an intervention, and quantitatively test whether it causes an effect (Shadish, Cook, & Campbell, 2002). A **mixed methods experiment** is a research design in which researchers embed qualitative methods within an experimental design to enhance the application of the experiment for determining the effects of an intervention. As alluded to in this definition, many of the writings about mixed methods experiments come from the perspective of embedding (or "adding") qualitative methods within an experimental design (e.g., Cooper et al., 2014; Creswell, Fetters, Plano Clark, & Morales, 2009; Drabble, O'Cathain, Thomas, Rudolph, & Hewison, 2014; Miller & Crabtree, 2005; Plano Clark et al., 2013), although there are a few who consider this design more from the perspective of mixing methods within the experimental design (e.g., Howe, 2004; Song, Sandelowski, & Happ, 2010). Examples of reasons that researchers add qualitative methods to experiments include improving experimental procedures (e.g., recruitment), examining implementation and fidelity issues, and understanding participants' perspectives and experiences with the intervention. A notable challenge associated with this approach is designing the use of qualitative methods so that they provide good qualitative information without introducing confounding issues and bias into the experimental controls.

Lin, Liu, and Chu (2011) employed an embedded quasi-experimental design to study the effect of in-class student use of "clickers" for promoting change in students' understanding of physics concepts in Taiwan. Their primary aim was to quantitatively determine whether the clickers caused positive outcomes in terms of students' learning, and they used a quasi-experiment to compare students in classes that used the clickers with those that did not in terms of their performance on posttest questions. The researchers carefully controlled the parameters of the experiment through decisions such as matching the amount of instructional time on topics across the classrooms and using a pretest of prior knowledge as a covariate in their analyses. Lin and colleagues embedded qualitative nonparticipant observation and interview methods within this experiment to examine students' behaviors and reactions in response to the treatment condition (use of clickers). They designed the qualitative methods carefully (e.g., scheduling interviews after completion of the posttest) so as to not introduce bias into the quantitative results. They used the qualitative findings to describe the treatment implementation and provide context to help explain why significant differences occurred in terms of students' conceptual learning but did not occur in terms of students' performance on basic calculations.

Mixed Methods Case Study

Case studies (including multiple case studies) can be defined as qualitative research designs in which researchers implement an in-depth exploration to describe and interpret what is happening in a bounded system, or case (Creswell, 2013; Stake, 1995; Yin, 2014). A **mixed methods case study** is a research design in which researchers embed quantitative methods within a case study design to enhance the application of the case study for examining the case(s). Scholars writing about mixed methods case studies approach them using one of two of the perspectives depicted in Figure 6.2: (a) intersecting by embedding or (b) intersecting by mixing methods within the case study approach. Across these two perspectives, mixed methods case studies are described as useful frameworks for integrating multiple paradigms and approaches to understand a complex case (Luck, Jackson, & Usher, 2006), for enriching qualitative case descriptions with quantitative information (Curry & Nunez-Smith, 2015), and for engaging with the complexities within bounded systems (Singh, Milne, & Hull, 2012). Examples of reasons for adding quantitative methods to case studies include better descriptions of macro contexts, assessing theoretically relevant constructs from case participants, and validating researchers' interpretations about the case. Challenges associated with this approach include designing the use of quantitative methods to provide useful information even with very small sample sizes and incorporating quantitative results in a meaningful way within rich case descriptions.

Bush and colleagues (2011) employed a mixed methods multiple case study design to study the complexity of the use of study skills for college students with severe traumatic brain injury. The researchers studied four cases to develop an in-depth understanding of each case. They gathered open-ended interviews with the selected students and key individuals associated with each of them (such as family members, advisors, and peers) as the primary qualitative data sources. They supplemented the interview data with field notes and student artifacts. To aid in their description of the focal students' study skills, the researchers employed a standard quantitative instrument for measuring college students' use of study skills and gathered quantitative data using the instrument from the focal students and from their peers. Using graphical displays and visual inspection analytic techniques, the researchers used the quantitative information to enrich their understanding of each of the focal students' study skills, including important differences in the perceptions held about them by different individuals.

Mixed Methods Evaluation

Evaluation includes a broad class of applied research approaches used to make judgments (such as about quality, value, or worth) about programs and policies (Patton, 2008; Rossi, Lipsey, & Freeman, 2004). A **mixed methods evaluation** is a research approach in which researchers integrate quantitative and qualitative methods within an evaluation methodological approach to enhance the application of this approach for addressing the evaluation goals. This design has also been referred to as a *mixed methods multiphase* (or *multistage*) *evaluation design* (Creswell 2015; Nastasi et al., 2007). Extensive writings exist that discuss mixed methods approaches to conducting evaluation research (e.g., Bamberger et al., 2010; Greene & Caracelli, 1997a; Nastasi et al., 2007; Nastasi & Hitchcock, 2016; Rallis & Rossman, 2003). Together, these writings emphasize the need for evaluators to intersect mixed methods with evaluation approaches to best address multiple questions; to satisfy diverse stakeholders; and to consider the multiple, complex facets associated with all programs and policies. The use of mixed methods within evaluation provides evaluators with the means to conduct rigorous needs assessment, theory development and adaptation, program development and testing, and ongoing monitoring while taking into account issues such as evaluating both process and impacts, considering cultural appropriateness, and acknowledging the complexity and multidimensionality of most important constructs targeted by programs and policies. Primary challenges associated with this approach include the extensive time, costs, and expertise required to carry out a multistage mixed methods evaluation and the difficulty of integrating diverse methods when they aim to address different questions or objectives.

Peterson and colleagues (2013) reported on their mixed methods multiphase evaluation approach to develop, refine, and test a theoretically informed behavior change intervention program aimed at increasing physical activity in populations with chronic illnesses. They implemented three specific phases of the project that lasted about 4.5 years and included over 1,000 participants in total. The first qualitative phase explored participants' values and beliefs about living with chronic illness. The team used the results from the qualitative phase to create culturally relevant materials, design components of the intervention, and inform the recruitment strategies for the pilot phase. The second mixed methods pilot phase iteratively examined and refined the intervention procedures. The mixed methods results from the pilot phase were used to revise aspects of the intervention and the associated methodologies as well as to ensure that the materials and procedures were culturally appropriate. In the final quantitative phase, the team tested the efficacy of the intervention for three specific populations using a quantitative experiment.

Mixed Methods Action Research

Action research is a methodological approach in which practitioners and researchers engage in a cyclical process to identify and take action to solve a practical problem in one's own practices or community (Hinchey, 2008; Reason

& Bradbury, 2008). Action research encompasses a wide variety of approaches, including *practitioner-based approaches* and *community-based participatory research* (CBPR). **Mixed methods action research** is a research approach in which researchers integrate quantitative and qualitative methods within an action research methodological approach to enhance the application of action research for solving the practical problem of interest. Discussions about mixed methods action research emphasize how a mixed methods way of thinking or doing can be applied within the cyclical stages of action research, including planning, acting, monitoring, and reflecting (Christ, 2009, 2010; Ivankova, 2015; Phillips & Davidson, 2009). These authors emphasize the compatibility of mixed methods research and action research in terms of the foundations, goals, and methods of these two forms of research. Ivankova (2015) advanced a mixed methods methodological framework for action research that illustrates how mixed methods or some procedural and conceptual aspects of it can be applied at each phase within an action research cycle. Although action research has been primarily associated with qualitative methods, the use and integration of qualitative and quantitative methods allows researchers to gather information that is more comprehensive and useful for guiding reflection and informing and monitoring action. Notable challenges with intersecting mixed methods and action research include navigating the integration of multiple methods throughout the cyclical action research process, including practitioners and community members as co-researchers, and designing the methods to be accessible and usable without becoming too cumbersome.

Greysen, Allen, Lucas, Wang, and Rosenthal (2012) used a mixed methods action research approach in their collaborative work to improve transitions from hospitals to shelters for individuals who are homeless. Before formally initiating the study, the first author engaged extensively with community members by attending meetings in the community and serving as a volunteer clinician in a shelter. Through this engagement, the problem of transitions from hospitals was identified as most important for this community and the first action plan was put into place to collect patient-centered data from individuals needing shelter in the community to learn more about their needs from their perspective. The collaborative team gathered quantitative and qualitative data from individuals staying at the shelter, integrated the two data forms during the analysis, and shared the results of their analysis with study participants and community stakeholders. From the sharing of the combined results, recommendations were developed and specific actions were implemented in the community to improve patients' transitions from a hospital to a homeless shelter.

Transformative Mixed Methods Research

Transformative theories, also referred to as transformative–emancipatory or social justice theories, are theoretical frameworks that challenge existing social power structures that marginalize and oppress certain groups (Mertens, 2003). Examples of such theories include, but are not limited to, gender theories, racial and ethnic theories, queer theories, and disability theories. **Transformative mixed methods research** is a research approach in which researchers explicitly integrate quantitative and qualitative methods within a social justice theoretical framework to enhance the application of research for addressing a social justice agenda. This type of mixed methods approach derives from the perspective of mixing methods within a theoretical framework. Key writers about this approach emphasize that researchers using this design base all of their study decisions in the core assumptions of their theoretical framework (Caracelli & Greene, 1997; Creswell, 2015; Hesse-Biber, 2010a; Mertens, 2003; Mertens et al., 2010; Sweetman, Badiee, & Creswell, 2010). The design decisions are directly shaped by the agenda to uncover and challenge social injustices and influence all stages of the research process, including problem identification; literature searching; quantitative and qualitative methods; and integrating, reporting, and using the results, to name only a few. Challenges associated with transformative mixed methods research include designing methods that refrain from reinforcing existing power imbalances (such as by not choosing a standard instrument developed for majority of individuals because it may not adequately represent the experiences of those who are marginalized), meaningfully integrating the methods within the theoretical framework, and using the research to bring about needed change.

McClelland (2014) used a feminist theoretical framework to approach her study topic of sexual satisfaction. Her assumptions included the existence of gendered norms related to sexuality, the importance of sociopolitical contexts of sexuality, and the heterogeneity of individuals' sexuality. These assumptions shaped all aspects of her transformative mixed methods design, which was conducted to include and differentiate perspectives across individuals who have different access to power within the sexual domain. To best understand and challenge assumptions about individuals' definitions of sexual satisfaction, McClelland used integrated methods proven to align well with feminist research goals, including a quantitative Q methodology to prioritize a wide range of existing perspectives about sexual satisfaction and qualitative in-depth interviews to better understand the nuances of individuals' personal definitions. She described each of her methods' decisions in terms of her feminist stance. The integrated results advanced several dimensions of sexual satisfaction that encompassed this phenomenon from the perspective of a wide range of individuals who differed in important ways in terms of gender and sexual status.

ISSUES AND DEBATES ABOUT INTERSECTING MIXED METHODS WITH OTHER APPROACHES

As discussed in Chapter 5, consensus does not exist in the field of mixed methods regarding how best to describe and delineate the different mixed methods designs. Our intent in this chapter has been to highlight several important perspectives and common approaches in the literature about advanced applications of mixed methods designs, and it should not suggest that there is one accepted approach to this topic. Even with that caveat in mind, however, there are issues and debates within the broad perspectives we have discussed. Here, we introduce three issues that have been raised about mixed methods research intersecting with other approaches in the literature.

   1. What does embedding (or nesting) really mean? There are many writings about embedding as an important mixed methods approach (e.g., Caracelli & Greene, 1997; Creswell & Plano Clark, 2011; Greene, 2007) and many examples of published studies that researchers' classify as having used an embedded mixed methods design. Despite this prominence in the literature, not all mixed methods scholars agree about its importance or even what it is. Some key discussions of mixed methods designs do not include embedding as an important option (e.g., Teddlie & Tashakkori, 2009). Other scholars go further to question whether embedding makes sense as a mixed methods concept and whether it has any value for discussing mixed methods designs (e.g., Morse & Niehaus, 2009). Even among scholars who discuss this approach, there are notable disagreements. For example, some writings limit embedding to concurrent approaches (Bazeley, 2010; Greene, 2007) while others discuss its application to concurrent and/or sequential approaches (Creswell & Plano Clark, 2011). Therefore, you need to recognize this perspective when it appears in the literature but also plan to carefully define the meaning of this term if you use it in your research practice.

2. Are these designs really advanced applications of mixed methods designs or have researchers been mixing methods in other designs all along? Thinking about hybrid approaches for mixed methods as defined in this chapter is a fairly new perspective in the field of mixed methods research. On the one hand, many scholars view this as an expansion in the potential use of mixed methods whereas, on the other hand, other scholars may view this as a misappropriation of what researchers have been doing traditionally for a long time (Creswell, 2010; Maxwell, 2015; Morse & Niehaus, 2009). For example, ethnographers and case study researchers have routinely collected both qualitative and quantitative data, quantitatively oriented researchers have typically talked to some people about a topic when needing to develop an instrument, and evaluators and action researchers have always been open to combining methods. When applying the concept of advanced applications of designs while reading, reviewing, and using mixed methods, consider whether there is clearly a formal overall design/approach/framework that is shaping the decisions made about the mixed methods research process as well as whether there is meaningful integration of the quantitative and qualitative methods within this overall design/approach/framework.

3. Is a transformative theoretical framework really an overall approach to research or simply a purpose for research? There is consensus among mixed methods scholars about the utility and value of mixed methods research for addressing transformative and social justice research purposes. Ongoing debates center around whether mixing methods within a transformative framework constitutes its own particular transformative mixed methods approach or is simply one possible reason for conducting mixed methods research. For example, Teddlie and Tashakkori (2009) do not consider the use of a theoretical framework as a component of mixed methods designs. They wrote, "the pursuit of social justice is not a design choice; rather, it is *the reason* for doing the research, which supersedes design choice" (p. 140, italics in original). Other compilations of mixed methods designs, however, do consider mixing methods within a theoretical framework as an important consideration for describing mixed methods designs (Creswell & Plano Clark, 2011; Greene, 2007; Mertens, 2003; Mertens et al., 2010). You should keep in mind that there is not consensus on this issue and be aware of the different perspectives that you will likely encounter in the literature.

These questions highlight important issues and debates in the ongoing conversations about advanced applications of mixed methods designs.

The diverse opinions also highlight the need for scholars to clearly define their own perspectives about mixed methods designs and to identify the perspective used by others who write about and apply mixed methods research. These varying perspectives form the basis for the considerations we suggest for mixed methods research practice in the next section.

APPLYING ADVANCED APPLICATIONS OF DESIGNS IN MIXED METHODS RESEARCH PRACTICE

The conduct of research is complicated because researchers end up creating unique research designs for their studies through the many decisions they make (Crotty, 1998). That said, the discussion of designs in the literature, including those about basic and advanced mixed methods design applications, provide useful guides for considering the logic and decisions involved in most research studies. Mixed methods designs that intersect two or more approaches add to the possibilities and complexities of mixed methods research practice and provide an important dimension for understanding how researchers use mixed methods research. In Box 6.1, we provide some general advice for considering these issues when reading about, reviewing, and conducting mixed methods research.

Box 6.1

Advice for Applying Advanced Applications of Designs in Mixed Methods Research Practice

Advice for Reading/Reviewing Mixed Methods Studies and Methodological Discussions

- Keep in mind that mixed methods designs are complex and often do not fit neatly into a small number of discrete design categories. It is more important to focus on the overall logic of a mixed methods approach instead of focusing on selecting a specific design name.
- When reading about and reviewing advanced applications of mixed methods designs, identify the other research design, methodological approach, or theoretical framework that intersected with the use of mixed methods.

(Continued)

(Continued)

- Expect the other research design, methodological approach, or theoretical framework in a hybrid mixed methods approach to be a formal methodology or theory that has been discussed extensively in the research literature.
- Note how the authors defined the other research design, methodological approach, or theoretical framework and justified and explained the need for mixed methods to intersect with its use.
- Identify the basic mixed methods design that was implemented within the other research design, methodological approach, or theoretical framework.
- Assess the extent to which the authors' decisions about the study's mixed methods research process (e.g., research questions, methods, and inferences) were consistent with the other research design, methodological approach, or theoretical framework.
- Assess the extent to which the authors' use of a hybrid mixed methods approach aligned with the research purpose and rationale.

Advice for Proposing/Reporting/Discussing Mixed Methods Research

- Thoughtfully articulate the reasons that your study calls for mixed methods to intersect with another research design, methodological approach, or theoretical framework.
- Describe your overall hybrid mixed methods approach, including your perspective for how mixed methods can intersect with another approach (i.e., embedding, mixing methods within a methodological approach, or mixing methods within a theoretical framework).
- Demonstrate your knowledge about and expertise with the other research design, methodological approach, or theory and cite supporting literature.
- Consider the other research design, methodological approach, or theoretical framework as you make *all* decisions about your research process from the study research purpose and questions, to methods, to drawing inferences.
- Apply good mixed methods research practices associated with the basic mixed methods designs within the other research design, methodological approach, or theoretical framework.

When reading and reviewing mixed methods literature, it is useful to consider the possibility of researchers intersecting mixed methods research with other approaches. Although the idea of intersecting can be very intuitive in some situations (such as when a researcher adds a small qualitative component to a study's experimental design), in many situations it can be difficult to clearly define and identify intersecting in research practice. The key is to keep in mind that for the advanced applications of designs discussed in this chapter, the use of mixed methods intersects with another formal research design, methodological approach, or theoretical framework throughout the entire design and implementation of the mixed methods research process. This is conceptually different from a basic mixed methods design that uses a clear logic for integrating quantitative and qualitative methods within concurrent and sequential study strands. For example, if researchers combine results from a large-scale survey with findings from a small number of case studies, they are implementing a good basic concurrent mixed methods design. This is different from a situation where researchers design a study using a case study research design and choose to embed quantitative and qualitative methods within that design in order to develop rich case descriptions. As another example, researchers often suggest implications for practice and needed changes as part of their interpretations at the end of a mixed methods study, but those suggestions alone do not make the study transformative mixed methods research because they do not represent a formal theoretical framework that guided the study's agenda and research process. Therefore, when reading about or reviewing advanced applications of mixed methods designs, it is important to focus attention on the authors' identification and use of another formal research design, methodological approach, or theoretical framework throughout every stage of the mixed methods study.

Likewise, it is important to carefully consider the definition and application of hybrid mixed methods approaches in your own mixed methods research practice. When intersecting mixed methods with another approach, it is essential to carefully define that other approach and explain how and why it is used to shape the application of the mixed methods research process. When using an advanced application of a mixed methods design, you should consider the implications of the other research design, methodological approach, or theoretical framework throughout every stage of your mixed methods study and articulate those considerations clearly to your audience. The use of an advanced approach can expand the possibilities for using mixed methods to address important research questions, but that possibility can only be realized if the design is carefully planned, thoughtfully implemented, and clearly explained.

CONCLUDING COMMENTS

We conclude the chapter by offering some final summary comments organized by the learning objectives stated at the beginning of the chapter.

- **Describe advanced applications of mixed methods designs.** Advanced applications of mixed methods designs are hybrid approaches where researchers add an additional layer of complexity to the application of a basic mixed methods design. This added layer occurs when researchers intersect (i.e., embed or join) mixed methods research with another research design, methodological approach, or theoretical framework. The added complexity results because researchers need to consider and navigate additional sets of assumptions and logics beyond those associated with the basic mixed methods design. Intersecting mixed methods with other approaches expands the possibilities for mixed methods research.

- **Understand different perspectives about the ways in which mixed methods research can intersect with other research designs, methodological approaches, and theoretical frameworks.** There are three major perspectives about intersecting mixed methods with other approaches: embedding a secondary method within a primary quantitative or qualitative research design, mixing methods within an established methodological approach, and mixing methods within a formal theoretical framework.

- **Consider how several different advanced applications of mixed methods designs are used in research practice.** Scholars are discussing and using advanced applications of mixed methods designs in which mixed methods research intersects with a wide array of other methodologies and theories. The most common applications include mixed methods experiments, mixed methods case studies, mixed methods evaluation, mixed methods action research, and transformative mixed methods research.

APPLICATION QUESTIONS

1. Consider a traditional quantitative research design with which you are familiar (e.g., true experiment, quasi-experiment, single-subject design, or survey design). List three reasons why a researcher might want to embed a secondary qualitative method in that design. How might that qualitative method be planned so that it fits the parameters of the primary quantitative design? You might consider how participants would be selected, the number of participants, the data collection and analysis procedures, and the interactions between the participants and the researcher.

2. Consider a traditional qualitative research design with which you are familiar (e.g., case study, ethnography, grounded theory, or phenomenology). List three reasons why a researcher might want to embed a secondary quantitative method in that design. How might that quantitative method be planned so that it fits the parameters of the primary qualitative design? You might consider how participants would be selected, the number of participants, the data collection and analysis procedures, and the interactions between the participants and the researcher.

3. Locate a published example of one of the five prominent advanced applications of mixed methods designs introduced in this chapter from your area of interest. Identify the other design, approach, or framework and the basic mixed methods design used in the study. Write a paragraph that describes this study's research design using the perspectives highlighted in this chapter. Include a specific example of how the study's authors intersected mixed methods research with the other approach.

4. Pick one of the ongoing issues and debates about advanced applications of mixed methods designs highlighted in this chapter. State why you selected that issue, and discuss your reactions to this issue in terms of the perspectives introduced in this chapter. How might this issue apply in your own mixed methods research practice?

KEY RESOURCES

To learn more about the considerations, issues, and debates around mixed methods intersecting with other approaches and frameworks, we suggest you start with the following resources that discuss each of the five hybrid approaches highlighted in this chapter:

1. **Creswell, J. W., Fetters, M. D., Plano Clark, V. L., & Morales, A. (2009). Mixed methods intervention trials. In S. Andrew & E. J. Halcomb (Eds.),** *Mixed methods research for nursing and the health sciences* **(pp. 161–180). Hoboken, NJ: Wiley-Blackwell.**

   • In this chapter, Creswell and colleagues discussed a variety of reasons and ways that researchers embed, nest, or add qualitative methods within the conduct of experimental research designs. They also highlighted several examples of published studies that demonstrate mixed methods experiments in research practice.

2. **Luck, L., Jackson, D., & Usher, K. (2006). Case study: A bridge across the paradigms.** *Nursing Inquiry, 13*(2), 103–109.

   • In this article, Luck and colleagues discussed case study as an overarching methodological approach for conducting research, including an overarching approach for mixing methods. The authors provided a thoughtful introduction to the mixed methods case study approach.

*3. **Nastasi, B. K., Hitchcock, J., Sarkar, S., Burkholder, G., Varjas, K., & Jayasena, A. (2007). Mixed methods in intervention research: Theory to adaptation.** *Journal of Mixed Methods Research, 1*(2), 164–182.

   • In this article, Nastasi and colleagues described the value of using mixed methods evaluation approaches to develop and assess culturally appropriate programs and policies. Drawing from experiences in a multiphase project in Sri Lanka, the authors introduced the many different ways that they mixed methods within the context of evaluating culturally appropriate mental health interventions.

4. **Ivankova, N. V. (2015).** *Mixed methods applications in action research: From methods to community action.* **Thousand Oaks, CA: Sage.**

   • In this book, Ivankova intersected current thinking about mixed methods research and action research to consider the theory and practice of a mixed methods action research approach for addressing practical problems and taking action.

*5. Sweetman, D., Badiee, M., & Creswell, J. W. (2010). Use of the transformative framework in mixed methods studies. *Qualitative Inquiry, 16*(6), 441–454.

- In this article, Sweetman and colleagues reviewed the use of transformative mixed methods designs in published mixed methods studies. They identified 13 transformative mixed methods studies and examined the authors' practices in terms of Mertens' (2003) recommendations for transformative mixed methods research.

* The key resource is available at the following website: http://study.sagepub.com/planoclark.

SEVEN

HOW TO ASSESS MIXED METHODS RESEARCH?

CONSIDERING MIXED METHODS RESEARCH QUALITY

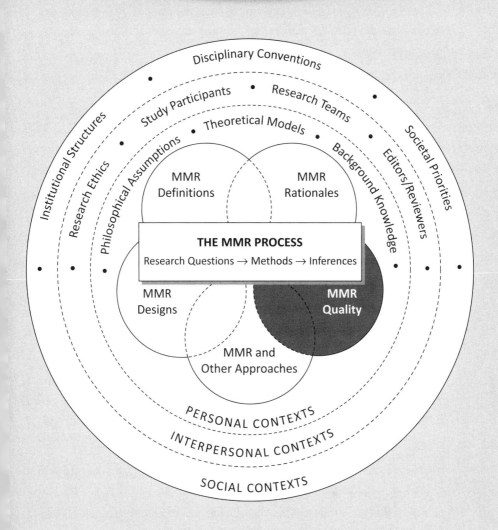

*N*ow that you have learned about basic and advanced applications of mixed methods designs, it is important to understand how to ensure that the inferences produced in a mixed methods study are of high quality and are credible. Quality assurance is an integral part of a mixed methods study and is another mixed methods research content consideration that directly influences the mixed methods research process. Multiple perspectives exist on what constitutes quality in mixed methods research and how to assess it. Knowing these perspectives will help you better understand the role that quality assurance plays in the design, conduct, and reporting of mixed methods studies. In this chapter, we describe a variety of perspectives about quality in mixed methods research and offer recommendations for how to assess quality of the mixed methods research process, including examples of quality assurance in mixed methods research practice.

LEARNING OBJECTIVES

This chapter aims to describe how to assess quality in mixed methods research so you are able to do the following:

- Understand the role of quality in the mixed methods research process.
- Recognize different perspectives about quality in mixed methods research.
- Understand how to assess quality in mixed methods research as it relates to study planning, implementation, reporting, and reviewing.

CHAPTER 7 KEY CONCEPTS

The following key concepts will help you navigate through the main considerations related to understanding quality in mixed methods research as they are introduced in this chapter:

- **Validation:** The process of assessing the rigor of the methodological procedures used in a study.
- **Mixed methods research quality:** The decisions that researchers have to make about how to assess and plan for quality of the mixed methods research process used in a study.
- **Validity:** The extent to which inferences can be accurately made based on test scores or other measures.
- **Reliability:** The extent to which the scores produced by a particular measurement procedure are consistent and reproducible.

- **Trustworthiness:** An umbrella term for quality in qualitative research that denotes the criteria that guide researchers in producing findings that can be accepted as persuasive and credible by others.
- **Credibility:** The extent to which the qualitative findings are perceived as accurately conveying the study participants' experiences.
- **Inference quality:** An umbrella term used to denote standards for evaluating the quality of conclusions that are made on the basis of research findings in a mixed methods study.
- **Inference transferability:** The degree to which conclusions from a mixed methods study can be applied to similar settings, contexts, and people.
- **Legitimation:** A process of continuous evaluation of all mixed methods study procedures for consistency between the research purpose and resulting inferences.

THE ROLE OF QUALITY IN THE FIELD OF MIXED METHODS RESEARCH

Quality assessment is a critical component of any research study because it makes the knowledge claims from the study more powerful and more representative of the problem under investigation (Koshy, Koshy, & Waterman, 2011). This process is often referred to as **validation** and implies assessing the rigor of the methodological procedures used in a study. The process of designing and conducting a mixed methods study goes hand in hand with assessing its quality and ensuring that the inferences produced in a study process are accurate. Therefore, we define *mixed methods research quality* as the decisions that researchers have to make about how to assess and plan for the quality of the mixed methods research process used in a study. For example, when you read or review a mixed methods study you have to think about whether it presents a good application of mixed methods research. You also consider mixed methods research quality when you weigh each methodological decision that goes into designing a mixed methods study's research process.

In mixed methods research, the process of assessing quality is complicated because of the need to collect, analyze, and mix two different data sets (Teddlie & Tashakkori, 2009). Researchers have to ensure that the inferences produced in the mixed methods research process are generated based on the application of sound quantitative and qualitative methods and are grounded in the credible findings from each study strand. However, what constitutes quality in mixed methods research may vary among different audiences—for example, academic journals, funding agencies, publishers, and teaching faculty. These differences reflect the many ways researchers approach quality in their mixed methods research practice when reading about, reviewing, conducting, and evaluating mixed methods research.

As we highlighted in our conceptual framework for mixed methods research and depicted in Figure 7.1, researchers' approaches to mixed methods quality and the frameworks or perspectives they use to guide their decisions

Figure 7.1 The Role of Quality in the Practice of Mixed Methods Research

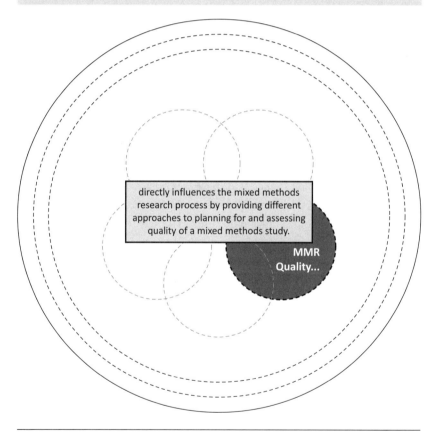

directly influences the mixed methods research process by providing different approaches to planning for and assessing quality of a mixed methods study.

MMR Quality...

NOTE: MMR = mixed methods research.

directly influence the mixed methods research process. These decisions are shaped by other mixed methods research content considerations (e.g., the rationale for using mixed methods research; the underlying logic of a mixed methods design) and the influences of the many factors that form researchers' personal, interpersonal, and social contexts. But before you can fully understand what constitutes quality in mixed methods research and the validation procedures, you need to recognize the different perspectives on this issue found in the mixed methods field.

MAJOR PERSPECTIVES ABOUT QUALITY FOR MIXED METHODS RESEARCH

The issue of quality in mixed methods research has long attracted mixed methods scholars; however, quality remains one of the major controversies in the mixed methods field (Creswell, 2015; Tashakkori & Teddlie, 2003a, 2010b), making it particularly complex to navigate. Scholars have different opinions of what counts as quality in mixed methods research (Bryman, Becker, & Semptik, 2008) and when quality should be assessed during the mixed methods research process (Creswell & Plano Clark, 2011). There are also observed paradigmatic differences in approaches to quality and quality standards used in mixed methods research (Bryman, 2006b; Giddings & Grant, 2009). That is, quality assessment standards and the choice of evaluation strategies are often influenced by researchers' philosophical views and epistemological practices that shape the terminology, definitions, and interpretations of quality in quantitative and qualitative research, and, consequently, the assessment of the quality of the integrated inferences in mixed methods research (Dellinger & Leech, 2007; Greene, 2007; Maxwell & Mittapalli, 2010). Across these different views and practices, three overarching perspectives about assessing quality are prominent in the mixed methods literature. Scholars discuss the need for assessing quality of the individual quantitative and qualitative study strands, evaluating quality of the generated inferences from an entire study, and also considering quality issues related to specific mixed methods designs.

Assessing Quality of Quantitative and Qualitative Study Strands

There is consensus among scholars that the quality of the respective quantitative and qualitative results directly affects the quality of the inferences drawn from an entire mixed methods study (Bryman et al., 2008; Creswell & Plano Clark, 2011; Dellinger & Leech, 2007; Greene, 2007; Onwuegbuzie & Johnson, 2006; Teddlie & Tashakkori, 2009). Failure to observe appropriate quality standards for the quantitative and qualitative methods used in a study might lead to a chain of erroneous conclusions resulting in less credible study outcomes. Indeed, Greene (2007) suggested differentiating between the quality of the quantitative and qualitative methods and related data used in the study as well as the quality of the mixed methods inferences produced from integrating those data. Therefore, as the first step in assessing quality of a mixed methods study, it is recommended to evaluate the quality of the data and the results in the quantitative and qualitative study strands using common quality standards adopted in quantitative and qualitative research (Creswell & Plano Clark, 2011; Curry & Nunez-Smith, 2015; Greene, 2007; Ivankova, 2014; Teddlie & Tashakkori, 2009).

There are different established criteria for assessing quality of data and results in quantitative and qualitative research. Traditional means for evaluating methodological quality of the quantitative data are to assess their validity and reliability using statistical procedures. **Validity** is defined as the degree to which inferences can be accurately made based on test scores or other measures, and **reliability** refers to the accuracy of measurement procedures to consistently produce the same scores (Thorndike & Thorndike-Christ, 2011). Validity is important in assessing the relevance of the collected data for answering the quantitative research questions, whereas reliability provides confidence that the same data will be collected using the same instruments to address similar research questions. A valid measure should always produce reliable data (Gay, Mills, & Airasian, 2012). Additionally, it is common to approach quantitative inference quality by assessing *internal* and *external* validity of the study results. Internal validity has to do with researchers' ability to draw correct inferences from the data, whereas external validity relates to the extent the study results can be generalized to a larger population.

In qualitative research, methodological quality of the data is assessed based on "whether the findings are accurate from the standpoint of the researcher, the participant, or the readers of an account" (Creswell, 2014, p. 201). In other words, researchers are interested in the trustworthiness and credibility of the qualitative findings and their interpretations. ***Trustworthiness*** is an umbrella term for quality in qualitative research that was introduced by Lincoln and Guba (1985). They defined *trustworthiness* broadly as the criteria that guide researchers in producing the findings that can be accepted as persuasive and "worth paying attention to" by others (p. 290). **Credibility** is one of the criteria of trustworthiness and refers to the extent to which the qualitative findings are perceived as accurately conveying the study participants' experiences. Strategies such as member checking, peer debriefing, data triangulation, and prolonged engagement are extensively used for ensuring quality of the qualitative findings. You can find further information about strategies for establishing quantitative validity and reliability as well as qualitative trustworthiness and credibility in some mixed methods books and articles (Creswell & Plano Clark, 2011; Dellinger & Leech, 2007; Onwuegbuzie & Johnson, 2006; Teddlie & Tashakkori, 2009) in addition to numerous research methods texts.

Assessing Quality of the Generated Inferences

As a second major perspective about mixed methods quality, many scholars emphasize the need to assess the degree to which the integration of the quantitative and qualitative methods in a mixed methods study produces quality inferences. Developing quality inferences that result from the mixing of quantitative and qualitative data sets is a critical point in the mixed methods research process and should be ongoing from the study design to results' interpretation. Recognizing the complex nature of quality assessment in mixed methods research, Teddlie and Tashakkori (2003) introduced the term *inference quality* as a criterion for considering quality of the generated inferences or *meta-inferences* as inductively and deductively derived conclusions from a mixed methods study. Inference quality is used with reference to "standards for evaluating the quality of conclusions that are made on the basis of research findings" in a mixed methods study (Teddlie & Tashakkori, 2009, p. 287). A related term is *inference transferability* that accounts for the degree a mixed methods study's conclusions can be applied to similar settings, contexts, and people (Teddlie & Tashakkori, 2009). Inferences that are of poor quality have no relevance and may be misleading for understanding the study outcomes.

Onwuegbuzie and Johnson (2006) suggested approaching mixed methods quality from the perspective of legitimation of the methods used and the inferences produced during the research process. They defined ***legitimation*** as a process of continuous evaluation of all mixed methods study procedures for consistency between the research purpose and resulting inferences. Considering the fundamental principle of mixed methods research that quantitative and qualitative methods should be integrated in a way that underscores their complementary strengths and nonoverlapping weaknesses, the authors warned about the legitimation threats that mixed methods researchers should be aware of "in obtaining findings and/or making inferences that are credible, trustworthy, dependable, transferable, and/or confirmable" (p. 52).

Dellinger and Leech (2007) introduced another perspective by comparing quality assessment in a mixed methods study with construct validity in quantitative research that embraces all validity evidence in a study. They viewed *construct validation* as "a continuous process of negotiation of meaning" that is created during the conduct of a mixed methods study (p. 320). Their approach to mixed methods validation focuses on exploring the meaning of the measures used in a mixed methods study and how these measures contribute to the quality and stability of the generated inferences.

Extending the idea of inference quality, Greene (2007) suggested a "multiplistic stance" in evaluating the quality of a mixed methods study (p. 167). This approach to judging mixed methods quality includes focusing on the support from the available data for the produced inferences, using criteria from different methodological traditions, encouraging dialogues among stakeholders about the generated inferences, and judging how a mixed methods study contributes to a better understanding of the studied problem.

All these perspectives highlight the importance of a rigorous approach to assessing the quality of the inferences produced as a result of the mixed methods research process used in a study. We will further discuss some of these approaches later in this chapter when we refer to the examples of mixed methods research quality from the methodological literature.

Assessing Quality Related to Specific Mixed Methods Designs

A third emerging perspective is found in discussions about quality as pertinent to specific features of mixed methods designs related to timing (concurrent or sequential) of the study strands and the integration of the quantitative and qualitative methods consistent with the purposes of the design. Curry and Nunez-Smith (2015) observed, "It is essential that the chosen study design is well suited to generate quantitative, qualitative, and integrated data that are directly relevant to answering the study question" (p. 183). Teddlie and Tashakkori (2009) suggested that criteria of quality related to design issues should include the following four indicators: (1) design suitability or appropriateness for answering the research questions, (2) design fidelity or adequacy of all study procedures, (3) within-design consistency of all components and study strands, and (4) analytic adequacy of data analysis procedures for answering the study's research questions. Creswell and Plano Clark (2007, 2011) linked a mixed methods study design, its characteristics, and the purposes of data integration with specific threats at the data collection, analysis, and interpretation levels that can compromise the quality of the produced inferences. Overcoming these threats is important for researchers to avoid inconsistent and wrongful conclusions caused by inadequate integration of quantitative and qualitative components within a mixed methods study.

In sequential designs, in which one study strand builds on another, the quality of the inferences produced in one study strand may markedly impact the quality of the inferences generated in another strand (Creswell & Plano Clark, 2011; Ivankova, 2014; Teddlie & Tashakkori, 2009). Ultimately, the quality of the inferences from an overall study may be affected due to a cumulative effect of inferences generated in each consecutive strand. The decisions about what research aspects to emphasize and what methodological strategies to use when connecting the study strands may either compromise or increase its quality. Ivankova (2014) advanced quality criteria in designing and conducting a sequential Quan → Qual mixed methods study, whereas Papadimitriou, Ivankova, and Hurtado (2013) provided eight quality checks for the sequential implementation of the quantitative and qualitative components in this mixed methods design. These validity standards relate to methodological procedures specifically focusing on the systematic use of methods, validation strategies, follow-up sample selection, choice of results for follow-up, interaction of the study components, and formulation of the meta-inferences.

EXAMPLES OF QUALITY FOR MIXED METHODS RESEARCH

Due to the different perspectives on what constitutes quality in mixed methods research, various examples of how quality is addressed at both conceptual and application levels are found within the mixed methods literature. Methodologists writing about mixed methods have focused on developing conceptual frameworks for assessing quality of a mixed methods study to guide a study's validation process. Alternatively, researchers oftentimes describe their own approaches used for quality assurance. We examine these two different approaches to assessing quality in mixed methods research in the following sections.

Examples of Quality from the Methodological Literature

Heyvaert, Hannes, Maes, and Onghena (2013) analyzed 13 existing frameworks for assessing quality of published mixed methods studies and revealed three general sets of criteria included in these frameworks. These criteria relate to evaluating separately the methodological quality of the quantitative and qualitative strands of a study, addressing quality concerns related to the integration of the methods, and appraising the quality standards generic to any research study. In spite of some consistency across the included quality standards, the frameworks differ in how the authors view quality in mixed methods research and what specific methodological aspects or domains they consider in establishing the criteria or indicators of quality. We listed examples of five such frameworks along with our brief descriptions in Table 7.1. We purposefully included these frameworks because they are often cited in the mixed methods literature, and you may encounter them in your mixed methods research practice. We also provided our comments about each framework, including the disciplinary contexts, the authors' approach to developing the framework, and its practical value for researchers. You can use the information in the table to help recognize the framework names commonly used in the mixed methods literature, note the criteria the authors selected for assessing mixed methods quality and their practical value for researchers as well as to identify the primary source for learning more about any one specific framework.

Examples of Quality Applied to Mixed Methods Research Studies

The call for a parsimonious set of quality standards that can be applied to judge the rigor of the mixed methods research process remains prominent in the mixed methods field (Creswell & Plano Clark, 2011). Along with methodologists providing conceptual frameworks for assessing mixed methods quality, researchers have been developing and applying different approaches and

Table 7.1 Conceptual Frameworks for Assessing Quality in Mixed Methods Research

Conceptual Frameworks (Authors)	Quality Domains	Brief Descriptions of Quality Indicators	Comments
Legitimation model (Onwuegbuzie & Johnson, 2006)	• Sample integration • Inside-outside • Weakness minimization • Sequential • Conversion • Paradigmatic mixing • Commensurability • Multiple validities • Political	• These nine domains of quality focus on assessing the way researchers develop quality meta-inferences by using sampling procedures, balancing insiders' and observers' views, building on the strengths of each method, observing sequence of quantitative and qualitative strands, implementing data transformation procedures, mixing philosophical beliefs, explicating worldviews, employing rigorous validation procedures, and considering consumers' perspectives.	This framework: • is provided by the authors writing in the context of social and educational research. • is based on the assumption that quality assessment is a process of continuous evaluation of all study procedures for consistency between the research purpose and resulting inferences. • provides researchers with a framework for understanding the potential legitimation threats to anticipate and address during the research process.
Validation framework (Leech, Dellinger, Brannagan, & Tanaka, 2010)	• Foundational element • Elements of construct validation for quantitative, qualitative, and mixed research • Inferential consistency	• These five domains of quality focus on assessing researchers' control over their background knowledge about the topic; reliance on quantitative, qualitative, and mixed methods validation strategies; consistency between study design,	This framework: • is provided by the authors writing in the context of social and educational research. • is based on the perspective of construct validity used in quantitative research that embraces all validity evidence in a study.

(Continued)

Table 7.1 (Continued)

Conceptual Frameworks (Authors)	Quality Domains	Brief Descriptions of Quality Indicators	Comments
	• Utilization/historical element • Consequential element	measurement, and analysis; use of multiple measures; and relevance of the research process used in a study to social acceptability of generated consequences.	• provides researchers with a framework for exploring the meaning of the measures used in a mixed methods study and how these measures contribute to the quality and stability of the generated research inferences.

Integrative framework for inference quality (Teddlie & Tashakkori, 2009)	• Design quality
	  ○ Design suitability
	  ○ Design fidelity
	  ○ Within-design consistency
	  ○ Analytic adequacy
		• These four domains of quality focus on assessing a mixed methods study design and address its suitability to answer the research question, fidelity of the study procedures and methodological rigor, consistency of all research aspects of the study, and adequacy of analytic procedures.	This framework:
			• is provided by the authors writing in the context of social and behavioral research.
			• is based on the assumption that quality assessment should occur at both the study design and inference interpretation levels when developing meta-inferences from the entire study.

			• provides researchers with a framework for understanding how to reduce inconsistencies between quantitative and qualitative inferences and assess the degree to which meta-inferences are valid and credible.

	• Interpretive rigor
	  ○ Interpretive consistency
	  ○ Theoretical consistency
	  ○ Interpretive agreement
	  ○ Interpretive distinctiveness
	  ○ Integrative efficacy
	  ○ Interpretive correspondence
		• These six domains of quality focus on assessing the interpretive rigor of meta-inferences that are produced as overall study outcomes and address consistency with findings, theory, and previous research; with the research purpose; with inferences from each study strand; with other possible interpretations by scholars and study participants; and with distinctiveness of credible conclusions.	

Comprehensive framework for assessing quality of mixed methods research (O'Cathain, 2010)	• Planning quality • Design quality • Data quality • Interpretive rigor • Inference transferability • Reporting quality • Synthesizability • Utility	• These eight domains of quality focus on assessing quality during the stages in the study design (quality of planning), implementation (quality of design, data, and their interpretation), and dissemination (transferability of inferences, quality of reporting, addition to knowledge base, and practical utility).	This framework: • is provided by the author writing in the context of health sciences research. • is based on the synthesis of different approaches to mixed methods quality assessment and is structured around eight domains of quality transcending all study elements. • provides researchers with a common language for and guidance on how to assess the quality of resulting inferences, using a comprehensive set of criteria.

(Continued)

Table 7.1 (Continued)

Conceptual Frameworks (Authors)	Quality Domains	Brief Descriptions of Quality Indicators	Comments
Critical appraisal framework for quality in mixed methods studies in health sciences (Curry & Nunez-Smith, 2015)	• Study conceptualization and justification • Design quality • Adherence to respective standards for qualitative and quantitative methods • Adherence to standards for mixed methods data analysis • Quality of analytic integration • Quality of interpretation	• These six domains of quality focus on assessing the rationale for using mixed methods; the choice of mixed methods design for addressing the research questions; methods for quantitative and qualitative sampling, data collection, and analysis; procedures for comparing and contrasting results; the appropriateness of the results' integration plan; and quality of the generated inferences.	This framework: • is provided by the authors writing in the context of health sciences research. • is based on the synthesis of different approaches to mixed methods quality appraisal and is structured around six broad domains of quality that relate to a mixed methods study design and conduct. • provides researchers with a set of minimum essential elements for assessing quality of mixed methods studies in the health sciences.

standards of research quality in their mixed methods research practice. These standards vary depending on researchers' personal and social contexts, such as their philosophical views, methodological perspectives, and discipline orientation (Bryman, 2006b; Creswell & Plano Clark, 2011; Maxwell & Mittapalli, 2010; O'Cathain, 2010). Additionally, different quality standards existing in quantitative and qualitative research contribute to differences in perceptions on how to assess the quality of the quantitative and qualitative components in a mixed methods study (Bryman et al., 2008). As a result, some researchers give more emphasis to assessing the quality of the methods used in a study, while some focus on the quality of the entire research process and its outcomes, whereas others emphasize the study design components. In each case, however, the focus is on validating the research aspects of the study to ensure the quality of the produced inferences.

Despite this plethora of views, quality criteria have been advanced for different types of mixed methods research practice that focus on designing, conducting, reporting, and reviewing mixed methods research. We summarized some of these criteria from different sources as applied to these research practices in Table 7.2. As expected, some of the existing criteria transcend across research practices making the criteria applicable to guiding both the mixed methods research process and its evaluation. The table highlights different sources including a methodological text, journal articles, journal editorial board guidelines, and a funding agency report. We also included our comments about each set of criteria, consisting of the disciplinary contexts, the authors' methodological orientation, and applicability of the quality criteria to types of mixed methods research practice. We recommend that you select and carefully review the criteria relevant to your mixed methods research practice wherever you evaluate the work of other researchers or prepare your own work for peer review.

ISSUES AND DEBATES ABOUT QUALITY IN MIXED METHODS RESEARCH

With many existing perspectives on what constitutes quality in mixed methods research, quality assessment remains one of the provocative methodological issues and most debatable topics in the mixed methods field (Teddlie & Tashakkori, 2010). As we highlighted in this chapter, the mixed methods literature

Table 7.2 Examples of Quality Standards Applied to Mixed Methods Research Practice

Mixed Methods Research Practice	Publication	Quality Criteria/Standards	Comments
Designing and implementing mixed methods research studies	*Designing and Conducting Mixed Methods Research* (Creswell & Plano Clark, 2011)	Researchers should do the following: • Collect both quantitative and qualitative data. • Employ rigorous data collection and analysis procedures. • Integrate different sources of data to better understand the research problem. • Use a mixed methods research design and integration strategies consistent with the design. • Use research terms adopted in the mixed methods field.	These quality criteria: • were developed by the authors writing in the context of social and behavioral research. • emphasize the methods used in a study. • can be used to guide both the mixed methods research process and its evaluation.
	Using Mixed Methods Research in Medical Education: Basic Guidelines for Research (Schifferdecker & Reed, 2008)	Researchers should do the following: • Identify the study design as mixed methods. • Decide on the weight of each data type in data collection, analysis, and results.	These quality criteria: • were developed by the authors writing in the context of health sciences research.

	• Develop sampling strategies to secure adequate and rigorous data. • Decide on data collection, analysis, and integration strategies. • Identify realistic timeframes for each project phase. • Use a software program to integrate quantitative and qualitative data. • Identify exemplary mixed methods articles for reporting results and displaying data.	• emphasize the study design components. • can be used to guide both the mixed methods research process and its evaluation.
Reporting mixed methods research	*Guidance for Good Reporting of a Mixed Methods Study (GRAMMS)* (O'Cathain, Murphy, & Nicholl, 2008)	Manuscripts should meet the following criteria: • Justify the use of mixed methods to address the research question. • Describe the design in terms of purpose, priority, and timing of each method. • Describe sampling, data collection, and analysis. • Explain methods' integration and limitations of each method. • Discuss any insights gained from mixing methods.	These quality criteria: • were developed by the authors writing in the context of health sciences research. • emphasize the study research process. • can be used to guide researchers in developing high-quality reports for mixed methods studies.

(Continued)

Table 7.2 (Continued)

Mixed Methods Research Practice	Publication	Quality Criteria/Standards	Comments
	Journal of Mixed Methods Research (JMMR)	Manuscripts that report empirical mixed methods research should meet the following criteria: • Fit the definition of mixed methods research by collecting and analyzing data, integrating the findings, and drawing inferences using both qualitative and quantitative approaches or methods. • Explicitly integrate the quantitative and qualitative aspects of the study. • Discuss how the work adds to the literature on mixed methods research in addition to making a contribution to a substantive area in the scholar's field of inquiry. Manuscripts that discuss methodological/theoretical issues of mixed methods research should meet the following criteria: • Address an important mixed methods topic. • Adequately incorporate existing literature. • Contribute to our understanding of mixed methods research.	These quality criteria: • were developed by the JMMR editorial board representing scholars from the social, behavioral, and health sciences. • emphasize adherence to the JMMR definition of mixed methods research. • provide guidelines for the authors in developing high-quality empirical and methodological mixed methods articles.

Reviewing mixed methods research	Journal of Mixed Methods Research (JMMR)	Manuscripts that report empirical mixed methods research should meet the following criteria: <ul><li>Describe noteworthiness of the problem, and the theoretical framework, and fit of questions to mixed methods design.</li><li>Discuss mixed methods design, sampling, methods for analysis, and integration.</li><li>Demonstrate insightfulness of discussion, quality of conclusions, and overall writing quality.</li><li>Explain contribution to mixed methods literature and interest to JMMR readership.</li></ul> Manuscripts that discuss methodological/ theoretical issues of mixed methods research should meet the following criteria: <ul><li>Address an important topic.</li><li>Adequately incorporate existing literature.</li><li>Provide soundness of the argument and originality of the suggestions.</li><li>Demonstrate writing quality.</li><li>Contribute to our understanding of mixed methods research.</li><li>Be of interest to JMMR readership.</li></ul>	These quality criteria: <ul><li>were developed by the JMMR editorial board representing scholars from the social, behavioral, and health sciences.</li><li>emphasize adherence to the JMMR definition of mixed methods research.</li><li>provide guidelines for reviewers in evaluating the quality of empirical and methodological mixed methods manuscripts.</li></ul>

(Continued)

Table 7.2 (Continued)

Mixed Methods Research Practice	Publication	Quality Criteria/Standards	Comments
	Best Practices for Mixed Methods Research in the Health Sciences (Creswell, Plano Clark, & Smith for the Office of Behavioral and Social Sciences Research, 2011)	Application for research funding should meet the following criteria: • Make a convincing case that the problem can best be studied using mixed methods, that the investigator(s) have the required research skills, that project leadership have commitment to mixed methods, and that collaboration is in place. • Demonstrate relevance of mixed methods for innovative investigation of the research problem(s), the philosophy or theory informing the research, the design suitability for the study aims, and innovative combination and integration of the methods. • Provide a clear description of the study design and methods' integration, including the timing, techniques, and responsible personnel; criteria for assessing rigor of quantitative and qualitative data collection and analysis; and computer software for each analytic component. • Demonstrate the study feasibility in terms of time and resources and evidence of the institution support for mixed methods.	These quality criteria: • were developed by the authors writing in the context of the health and social sciences. • are part of the recommendations for using mixed methods research in the context of grant applications to the NIH. • emphasize an overall quality of applications for research funding for R series grant awards. • can be used to guide both researchers in developing the applications and reviewers in evaluating the applications.

offers a number of conceptual models and frameworks for assessing quality that include different components, use different language, and focus on different procedural issues. You should be aware of these differences in existing approaches to be able to make informed decisions when planning for and assessing quality of mixed methods studies in your own research practice. Here, we introduce some of the issues about quality in mixed methods research that continue to be discussed and debated within the field of mixed methods research.

1. Should we use a common language related to quality in mixed methods research? There is ongoing debate about what terminology is best to use when discussing quality considerations in mixed methods research. Lack of common understanding of what constitutes quality in mixed methods by scholars from quantitative and qualitative research traditions has resulted in the existence of different terms that are used to discuss mixed methods research quality (Creswell, 2010; O'Cathain, 2010; Teddlie & Tashakkori, 2003, 2010). Some scholars focus on the quality of the collected data and approach quality assessment from the position of individual quantitative and qualitative approaches using the terms adopted in these research traditions, such as *validity, reliability, credibility,* etc. (Bryman et al., 2008). Others emphasize the quality of inferences that are the outcome of the analysis of the quantitative and qualitative data sets and refer to their quality using either existing terms similar in meaning, such as *construct validity* (Dellinger & Leech, 2007) or create terms unique to mixed methods research, such as *inference quality* (Teddlie & Tashakkori, 2003) and *legitimation* (Onwuegbuzie & Johnson, 2006). At the same time, the term *validity* was suggested as a generic term for mixed methods quality because of its use in both quantitative and qualitative research (Creswell & Plano Clark, 2011; Maxwell & Mittapalli, 2010). Whatever term you select to refer to mixed methods research quality should be justified and supported by relevant literature.

2. Should we have standards to assess the quality of a mixed methods study? Creswell (2015) reviewed the pros and cons of applying quality standards for mixed methods research and provided several compelling reasons justifying their need along with the argument about their restricting role. For example, standards are useful in evaluating the quality of mixed methods journal manuscripts, conference papers, proposals for funding, and graduate students' theses and dissertation projects to ensure consistency among the reviewers in appraising the work and providing their feedback. Similarly, standards are seen as more useful and necessary in disciplines with a heavy quantitative orientation, such as the health sciences and where the use of valid standardized instruments is encouraged. At the same time, standards may restrict researchers' ability to apply mixed methods in new creative ways and eventually "slow down the adoption of mixed methods" (Creswell, 2015, p. 101). Additionally standards may have a degree of bias, as they are the product of human beings approaching mixed methods from their own philosophical, political, and knowledge backgrounds. However, if you are new to mixed methods or experimenting with mixed methods in new ways, having quality standards will help you produce credible mixed methods research outcomes.

3. When should quality be assessed in the mixed methods research process? There are debates in the mixed methods literature about when quality should be assessed during a mixed methods study conduct and whether an additional set of quality standards is needed beyond those advanced in quantitative and qualitative research. Some scholars focus on the quality of the collected data and approach quality assessment from the position of individual quantitative and qualitative study components (Bryman et al., 2008), whereas others adopt a more holistic or framework approach and emphasize the need for a separate set of criteria embracing an entire mixed methods research process and its outcomes (Onwuegbuzie & Johnson, 2006; Teddlie & Tashakkori, 2009). There are also discussions related to whether only a completed study should be evaluated for quality or if quality assessment should begin as early as the study proposal phase (O'Cathain, 2010). You need to carefully consider all these views when approaching quality assessment in your own mixed methods research practice.

These three questions highlight important issues and debates related to quality assessment in mixed methods research. They also indicate the importance for researchers to identify and recognize their own approaches to assessing quality of their mixed methods studies in order to ensure the produced inferences are accurate and credible.

APPLYING QUALITY IN MIXED METHODS RESEARCH PRACTICE

As we have shown, assuring quality of a mixed methods study has important implications for the quality of the inferences produced as a result of the research process. The ability to plan for and assess quality in a mixed methods study is equally important for reading and reviewing mixed methods research done by others as well as for proposing and reporting your own mixed methods project. Box 7.1 includes our advice for applying the concepts of this chapter to your mixed methods research practice.

When reading and reviewing the literature about mixed methods research, it is essential to pay particular attention to how researchers assessed quality in

---

Box 7.1

Advice for Applying Quality Considerations in Mixed Methods Research Practice

Advice for Reading/Reviewing Mixed Methods Studies and Methodological Discussions

- When reading about and reviewing mixed methods studies, note what perspectives the authors emphasized in their approach to mixed methods quality and how these perspectives might be influenced by quality standards adopted in their disciplines.
- Identify if the authors explicitly discussed assessing quality of their mixed methods studies.
- Note what terms the authors used with reference to mixed methods quality and what literature they cited to support their choice of the terms.
- Note how the authors approached assessing quality in mixed methods research, such as by citing a certain quality framework or explaining the reasons for their approach.
- In reviewing a published mixed methods study, assess the extent the authors followed the quality criteria advanced by the journal.
- In reviewing a grant application for a mixed methods study, assess the extent the authors adhered to the quality standards adopted by the funding agency.
- In reviewing a student's proposal for a mixed methods study, assess the extent the author adhered to the quality standards suggested by the program and supervisory committee.

(Continued)

(Continued)

Advice for Proposing/Reporting/Discussing Mixed Methods Research

- Start thinking about how to ensure mixed methods research quality early during the study planning and designing stages.
- Explain your approach to ensuring mixed methods research quality, citing supporting mixed methods literature.
- Choose a term to refer to mixed methods research quality that aligns best with your epistemological practices; explain the term and provide supporting references from the mixed methods literature.
- Choose a framework for assessing mixed methods research quality, and justify your selection using supporting mixed methods literature.
- Describe how you plan to ensure or ensured the quality of the quantitative and qualitative study strands and the inferences generated from an entire study.
- Note and address the quality issues related to specific mixed methods designs (concurrent and sequential).
- Closely adhere to the suggested quality standards when you prepare a journal manuscript reporting a mixed methods study, a grant application for a mixed methods research project, or a thesis and dissertation proposal for a mixed methods study.

their mixed methods studies. As we have explained, the major perspectives on assessing quality in mixed methods research along with the quality standards prominent in different disciplines might influence how researchers apply quality criteria in their mixed methods research practice. More specifically, researchers may use different terms with reference to mixed methods quality, adopt different frameworks for assessing quality, and apply different standards and quality criteria to the mixed methods research process. So it is important to note if researchers explicitly discussed assessing quality of their mixed methods studies and what mixed methods literature they cited to justify and support their approaches. Depending on the purposes of your engagement with mixed methods, pay close attention to how researchers adhered to the quality

standards suggested by the journals, funding agencies, and thesis and dissertation committees. Assessing the degree of adherence to these standards may
help you evaluate the quality of the reported mixed methods research process
and the produced inferences.

It is equally important to adhere to rigorous standards when designing,
conducting, and reporting your own mixed methods study. Strategies to ensure
a mixed methods study's quality should be included in the study design plan and
ensuring quality should be an ongoing process. Readers who will review and
evaluate your study will benefit if you clearly articulate your approach to ensuring mixed methods research quality and the selection of terms and frameworks.
Always support your choice by citing relevant mixed methods literature. In
addition, describe how you ensure the quality of the quantitative and qualitative
study strands and address the quality issues related to specific mixed methods
designs (concurrent and sequential). Finally, closely adhere to the appropriate
quality standards such as those advanced by the journal, funding agency, and
your thesis or doctoral dissertation committee. By fully explaining your
approach to ensuring mixed methods research quality, readers will be in a better
position to understand and evaluate your mixed methods research practice.

CONCLUDING COMMENTS

We conclude the chapter by offering some final summary comments organized
by the learning objectives stated at the beginning of the chapter.

- **Understand the role of quality in the mixed methods research
  process.** Mixed methods research quality addresses decisions that
  researchers have to make about how to assess and plan for the quality of
  the mixed methods research process used in a study. In mixed methods
  research, the quality of the produced inferences is determined by the quality of the collected data and their analysis in each quantitative and qualitative study strand as well as the methods of data and results integration.
- **Recognize different perspectives about quality in mixed methods
  research.** Several perspectives and conceptual frameworks about
  assessing quality are prominent in the mixed methods literature.
  Scholars discuss assessing quality of the individual quantitative and
  qualitative study strands, evaluating quality of the generated inferences

from an entire study, and also considering quality issues related to specific mixed methods designs.

- **Understand how to assess quality in mixed methods research as it relates to study planning, implementation, reporting, and reviewing.** Along with conceptual frameworks for assessing quality in mixed methods research, quality criteria have been advanced for different types of mixed methods research practice. Some criteria transcend across these practices and are applicable to guiding both the mixed methods research process and its evaluation. Quality criteria may vary depending on scholars' philosophical views, methodological perspectives, and discipline orientation.

APPLICATION QUESTIONS

1. Reflect on the major perspectives about quality in mixed methods research discussed in this chapter. Discuss how these perspectives may shape your approach to assessing the quality of a mixed methods study. Explain why you think approaching the assessment of quality from a certain perspective or perspectives may be important and how this may influence your planning, conducting, reporting, and evaluating mixed methods research.

2. Examine the conceptual frameworks for assessing quality in mixed methods research presented in Table 7.1. Choose two frameworks, and compare and contrast the quality indicators that are included in these frameworks. Study our comments about these frameworks in Table 7.1, and describe the methodological aspects that the authors considered in selecting the indicators of quality.

3. Locate a mixed methods published study in your discipline or area of interest. Evaluate how the quality was assessed for each quantitative and qualitative study strand and the resulting inferences from the entire study. Pay particular attention to the quality standards and procedures for quality assessment reported in the study.

4. Choose one issue from the ongoing issues and debates about quality in mixed methods research: common language for mixed methods quality, standards for assessing a mixed methods study quality, and when

to assess quality in the mixed methods research process. State why you selected that issue, and discuss your reactions to it in terms of how this issue might affect your approach to planning for and assessing quality of mixed methods studies in your own research practice.

KEY RESOURCES

To learn more about quality in mixed methods research, we suggest you start with the following resources:

1. **Onwuegbuzie, A. J., & Johnson, R. B. (2006). The validity issue in mixed research.** *Research in the Schools, 13*(1), 48–63.

   - In this article, Onwuegbuzie and Johnson advanced nine types of legitimation as standards for assessing quality when combining inferences from the quantitative and qualitative components of the mixed methods study.

*2. **Heyvaert, M., Hannes, K., Maes, B., & Onghena, P. (2013). Critical appraisal of mixed methods studies.** *Journal of Mixed Methods Research, 7*(4), 302–327.

   - In this article, Heyvaert and colleagues analyzed available frameworks for evaluating quality of mixed methods published studies and compared the quality criteria included in these frameworks.

3. **O'Cathain, A. (2010). Assessing the quality of mixed methods research: Toward a comprehensive framework. In A. Tashakkori & C. Teddlie (Eds.),** *SAGE handbook of mixed methods in social & behavioral research* **(2nd ed., pp. 531–555). Thousand Oaks, CA: Sage.**

   - In this chapter, O'Cathain reviewed different conceptualizations of quality in mixed methods research and described a comprehensive framework for assessing quality of mixed methods research using eight domains.

4. **Curry, L., & Nunez-Smith, M. (2015). Assessing quality in mixed methods studies. In** *Mixed methods in health sciences research: A practical primer* **(pp. 169–200). Thousand Oaks, CA: Sage.**

- In this chapter, Curry and Nunez-Smith provided a comprehensive overview of issues of quality in mixed methods research and presented a critical appraisal framework for quality in mixed methods studies in the health sciences.

* The key resource is available at the following website: http://study.sagepub.com/planoclark.

PART III

CONTEXTS THAT SHAPE MIXED METHODS RESEARCH PRACTICE

We now turn our focus to the contexts that directly influence mixed methods research practice by shaping scholars' perspectives about mixed methods research content considerations and decisions about the mixed methods research process. The three contextual domains in our conceptual framework for mixed methods research represent the prominent types of contexts discussed in the field of mixed methods research. These discussions aim to unravel and describe the influences that researchers' beliefs and experiences, interactions with others, and disciplinary and societal environments have on the use of mixed methods research. In the chapters that follow, we present the major perspectives that exist for each research contextual domain, highlight important issues and debates among those perspectives, provide examples of how the perspectives influence the use of mixed methods research, and offer recommendations for considering the contexts in mixed methods research practice. The chapters in Part III are as follows:

EIGHT

HOW DO PERSONAL CONTEXTS
SHAPE MIXED METHODS?

*CONSIDERING PHILOSOPHICAL, THEORETICAL,
AND EXPERIENTIAL FOUNDATIONS
FOR MIXED METHODS RESEARCH*

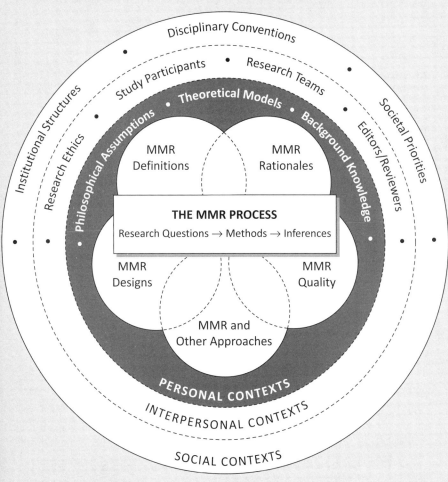

Now that we have introduced you to the major content considerations involved in the practice of mixed methods research, we are ready to consider the contexts that directly influence these research considerations. We start by discussing how scholars' personal contexts—such as their philosophical assumptions about knowledge, theoretical models about the study topic, and background knowledge and experiences—play an important role in how they think about and apply mixed methods research. All researchers bring their personal contexts with them to the process of research, and it is important to understand how different assumptions, theories, and backgrounds shape researchers' decisions about their mixed methods research practice. In this chapter, we discuss the role of personal contexts and introduce perspectives and debates related to these contexts for mixed methods research, including examples of addressing personal contexts in mixed methods research practice.

LEARNING OBJECTIVES

This chapter aims to provide you with an understanding of personal contexts that shape mixed methods research content considerations and research process so you are able to do the following:

- Understand different personal contexts for mixed methods research.
- Recognize how personal philosophical assumptions, theoretical models, and background knowledge provide foundations for mixed methods research practice.
- Describe different stances about personal contexts for mixed methods research.

CHAPTER 8 KEY CONCEPTS

The following key concepts will help you navigate through the main considerations related to personal contexts for mixed methods research as they are introduced in this chapter:

- **Mixed methods research contexts:** The circumstances, including beliefs, background, environment, framework, setting, relationships, and communities, that shape the practice of mixed methods research and in terms of which it can be fully understood and assessed.

- **Personal contexts:** The philosophical assumptions, theoretical models, and background knowledge that shape mixed methods research practice.
- **Philosophical assumptions:** Beliefs and values about the nature of reality, including how one is able to gain knowledge about that reality, that provide the philosophical foundation for mixed methods research practice.
- **Theoretical models:** Assumptions about the nature of a substantive topic, including how it works in the world, that provide the theoretical foundation for mixed methods research practice.
- **Background knowledge:** Personal and professional experiences and expertise, including substantive and methodological training and skills, that provide the experiential foundation for mixed methods research practice.

THE ROLE OF PERSONAL CONTEXTS IN THE FIELD OF MIXED METHODS RESEARCH

Recall our socio-ecological model for mixed methods research as introduced in Chapter 1. The outer layers of the model represent different domains of **mixed methods research contexts**, which we define as the beliefs, background, environment, framework, setting, relationships, and communities that shape the practice of mixed methods research and in terms of which it can be fully understood and assessed. We start by focusing on personal contexts, because they most directly guide researchers' decisions and actions and are themselves influenced by interpersonal and social contexts. **Personal contexts** are the philosophical assumptions, theoretical models, and background knowledge that shape mixed methods research practices. For example, you have philosophical assumptions about the kinds of knowledge that can and should be obtained through research and the role the researcher should take in that knowledge generation. You also have theoretical models in mind about the nature of the topic being studied and its connections with other related concepts and facts. You also bring your particular expertise and prior experiences related to the content topic and conducting research as important background knowledge. Taken together, these beliefs and experiences form the personal contexts for and provide the foundation of your use of mixed methods research (Greene, 2007).

Personal contexts play an important role in all research. As Maxwell and Mittapalli (2008) highlighted, a researcher's personal context is "an inescapable component of all research, whether or not it is explicitly acknowledged" (p. 877). Since personal contexts are so closely tied to researchers, they are often the contexts that most directly influence many of the decisions found within mixed methods research practice (see the dark shaded inner circle of Figure 8.1). Likewise, due to the personal nature of these contexts, they are also among the concepts that have evoked the most passionate and contentious debates in the field of mixed methods research (Greene & Caracelli, 1997a; Tashakkori & Teddlie, 1998). As Figure 8.1 highlights, personal contexts directly impact mixed methods research content considerations such as how researchers choose

Figure 8.1   The Role of Personal Contexts in the Practice of Mixed Methods Research

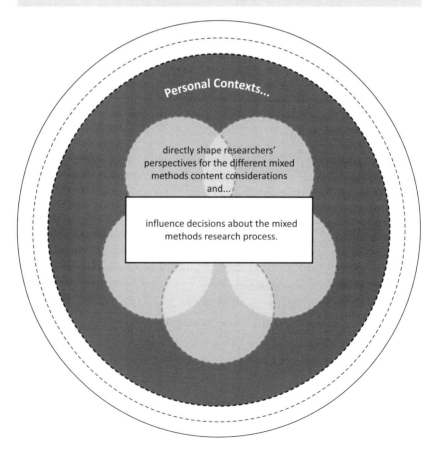

to define mixed methods research and their rationales for using mixed methods. In addition, personal contexts also directly influence researchers' decisions about the mixed methods research process (Maxwell & Loomis, 2003; Morgan, 2014; Onwuegbuzie, Frels, Collins, & Leech, 2013; Plano Clark & Badiee, 2010). For example, a particular theoretical stance may influence researchers' choice of research questions, and extensive training in a particular method may influence the priority of the quantitative and qualitative methods that research-ers use in their studies. Therefore, to fully understand mixed methods content considerations and the mixed methods research process, you need to account for how they are influenced and shaped by researchers' personal contexts.

MAJOR PERSPECTIVES ABOUT PERSONAL CONTEXTS FOR MIXED METHODS RESEARCH

Personal contexts are an essential consideration for all types of research approaches. The ways in which these contexts are considered, however, differ significantly across the different research approaches. On the one hand, litera-ture about quantitative research often emphasizes the importance of controlling and limiting the influence of personal contexts in order to achieve objectivity in research. On the other hand, scholars writing about qualitative research often emphasize the importance of acknowledging and reflecting about per-sonal contexts as essential and valued elements of a researcher's subjectivity in research. Divergent views such as these necessarily coexist in the field of mixed methods and contribute to a wide variety of perspectives for personal contexts in relation to the practice of mixed methods research. In the sections that follow, we view personal contexts as providing *foundations* for research because they are the fundamental basis from which researchers consider mixed methods research and make decisions about how to apply it. Building from several existing frameworks (e.g., Crotty, 1998; Greene, 2007; Maxwell, 2013), we discuss these foundations as three broad, interrelated categories: philosophical assumptions, theoretical models, and background knowledge.

Philosophical Assumptions

When researchers conduct research about a topic in the social and behav-ioral sciences, they operate with certain philosophical assumptions about what it means to do research. **Philosophical assumptions** are beliefs and values about the nature of reality, including how one is able to gain knowledge about that reality, that provide the philosophical foundation for a mixed methods research study. Philosophers and methodologists have articulated several formalized sets of philosophical assumptions (also referred to as *philosophies, worldviews,* and *paradigms*) and considered their implications for conducting research both in general and for mixed methods in particular. Examples of formal philosophies for research include positivism, postpositivism, constructivism, pragmatism, and postmodernism. Philosophies such as these are often distinguished in terms of beliefs about the nature of social reality (ontological assumptions), beliefs about how one can generate knowledge about that reality (epistemological assumptions), and beliefs about the role of values for learning about reality (axiological assumptions) (Crotty, 1998; Neuman, 2011).

To help illustrate these concepts, we first examine these different types of beliefs in the context of two well-known philosophies: postpositivism and constructivism. Postpositivism assumes that there is a single reality, that the researcher can best learn about that reality as a distant and independent observer, and that the researcher should try to control her or his values and remove their influence from the research as much as possible (Crotty, 1998; Tashakkori & Teddlie, 1998). Postpositivism has traditionally been viewed as providing a philosophical foundation for quantitative research aimed at measuring variables in order to make causal inferences and generalizations about reality. In contrast, constructivism assumes that each individual constructs her or his own reality and therefore there are multiple realities, that the researcher can only learn about these realities by constructing knowledge with individuals, and that a researcher's values cannot be separated from the research (Lincoln & Guba, 1985). Constructivism has traditionally been viewed as providing a philosophical foundation for qualitative research aimed at describing multiple realities through a reflexive process in order to interpret the meaning and contexts for individuals' experiences. Although many scholars emphasize that absolute links do not exist between certain philosophies and certain research methods (e.g., Greene, Caracelli, & Graham, 1989; Reichardt & Cook, 1979; Tashakkori & Teddlie, 1998), these two examples highlight how a researcher's assumptions (e.g., there is a single measurable reality *or* there are multiple constructed realities) can have salient implications for how research about the social world is conceptualized and implemented. These different views and their implications are especially important in the context of mixed methods research because researchers use and integrate different research approaches, thus potentially operating from and/or combining different philosophical assumptions within one study.

Table 8.1 identifies several philosophies that have received attention in the mixed methods literature along with brief descriptions of the assumptions associated with each one. In addition, the table highlights a selection of readings from the mixed methods literature that provides more detailed information about the key tenets for each philosophy. Several authors have also considered the implications of these different philosophies specifically for the practice of mixed methods research (Christ, 2013; Shannon-Baker, 2015). We provide some comments about these implications in the context of mixed methods research within the last column of the table. These comments should not be taken as absolutes but instead are intended as illustrations of possible ways that researchers' philosophical assumptions might influence decisions about mixed methods research. For example, a researcher's philosophical assumptions may influence her or his perspectives about the different mixed methods research content considerations, such as defining mixed methods in terms of a method, methodology, philosophy, or community or the choice to intersect mixed methods with another design, approach, or framework. Likewise, these assumptions may influence the mixed methods research process, such as the priority attributed to the methods or the meaning of integration within the context of the study.

Theoretical Models

Scholars bring more than philosophical assumptions about reality to their mixed methods research practice. They also bring theoretical models that inform their approach to the substantive topic of interest. **Theoretical models** are assumptions about the nature of a substantive topic, including how it works in the world, that provide the theoretical foundation for mixed methods research practice. Theoretical models range from very broad theoretical frameworks (e.g., feminist theory, critical race theory, and complexity theory) to middle-range theories (e.g., self-determination theory, theory of self-efficacy, and theory of planned behavior) to specific hypotheses (e.g., more time on task causes better math performance). An illustration of using a theoretical model is our use of the socio-ecological theory (introduced in Chapter 1) in this book to guide our assumptions about how mixed methods research practice works. Based on this model, we made assumptions about the key elements (i.e., the

Table 8.1 Examples of Prominent Philosophies Discussed in the Mixed Methods Literature

Philosophy	Brief Description of the Ontological, Epistemological, and Axiological Assumptions[1]	Selected Mixed Methods Writings	Comments
Postpositivism	• There is a single reality. • Knowledge about reality is obtained by being a distant and independent observer. • The influence of a researcher's values should be largely controlled and removed from the research.	• Giddings and Grant (2007) • Ridenour and Newman (2008) • Tashakkori and Teddlie (1998)	• This philosophy is the traditional foundation for quantitative research that measures variables in order to make causal inferences and generalizations about reality. • When used as the foundation for mixed methods, researchers often prioritize the quantitative methods, "quantitize" qualitative findings for statistical analysis, and emphasize causal inferences and generalizations. • Critics of this foundation for mixed methods research note how it tends to constrain the qualitative methods to more structured approaches.
Constructivism/ Interpretivism	• Individuals construct their own reality; therefore, there are multiple realities. • Knowledge about realities is constructed with individuals.	• Flick, Garms-Homolová, Herrmann, Kuck, and Röhnsch (2012) • Howe (2011) • Mason (2006)	• This philosophy is the traditional foundation for qualitative research that describes multiple realities through a reflexive process in order to interpret the meaning of and contexts for individuals' experiences.

	• A researcher's values and reflexivity cannot be separated from the research.		• When used as the foundation for mixed methods, researchers often prioritize the qualitative methods, limit the research to a small number of information-rich cases, and emphasize each researcher's reflexivity and interpretations. • Critics of this foundation for mixed methods research note how it tends to limit the quantitative methods to descriptive statistical analyses.
Pragmatism	• The viewpoints about reality are diverse. • Knowledge is gained through iterations of independent observations and subjective constructions. • The influence of a researcher's values are particularly important for stating the research questions and drawing conclusions.	• Biesta (2010) • Feilzer (2010) • Johnson and Onwuegbuzie (2004) • Morgan (2007)	• This philosophy is often advanced as providing a strong foundation for mixed methods research. • When used as the foundation for mixed methods, researchers emphasize the role of the research questions for directing methods decisions (i.e., using "what works") and the importance of the inferences drawn in response to those questions. • Critics of this foundation for mixed methods research note that it tends to minimize the epistemological differences between the quantitative and qualitative approaches and inadequately consider who gets to decide what works.

(Continued)

Table 8.1 (Continued)

Philosophy	Brief Description of the Ontological, Epistemological, and Axiological Assumptions[1]	Selected Mixed Methods Writings	Comments
Dialectical perspective/ Dialectical pluralism	• There are different ways to conceptualize reality. • Knowledge is enhanced through respectful dialogue among different conceptualizations. • Values of tolerance, acceptance, and equity are particularly important.	• Greene and Caracelli (2003) • Greene and Hall (2010) • Johnson (2012) • Onwuegbuzie and Frels (2013)	• This philosophical perspective is receiving increasing attention as providing a strong foundation for mixed methods research. • When used as the foundation for mixed methods, researchers tend to emphasize dialogue among different philosophical positions within a study, including examples of both convergence and divergence, in addition to or over methods-based considerations. • Critics of this foundation for mixed methods research note that it tends to overemphasize the epistemological differences between the quantitative and qualitative approaches and offers inadequate guidance for how to mix contradictory assumptions.
Transformative– emancipatory perspective	• There are multiple realities constructed through underlying socio-political structures.	• Biddle and Schafft (2014) • Mertens (2003; 2007) • Mertens, Bledsoe, Sullivan, and Wilson (2010)	• This philosophical perspective is advanced as providing a strong foundation for mixed methods research for individuals driven by social justice perspectives.

	• Knowledge about realities is gained through collaboration with individuals who experience them. • A researcher's values are an essential part of research, and some values are more moral than others.		• When used as the foundation for mixed methods, researchers tend to emphasize the use of mixed methods within a theoretical framework in order to advance a social justice agenda by challenging the status quo and working for change for individuals who have been marginalized. • Critics of this foundation for mixed methods research note that it tends to overemphasize values and that its social justice agenda is better considered a purpose for research than a philosophical assumption.
Critical realism	• There is a reality that includes the real world and mental phenomena. • Knowledge about reality is constructed from a researcher's particular perspective. • A researcher's values are part of the research.	• Maxwell and Mittapalli (2010) • Harrits (2011) • Zachariadis, Scott, and Barrett (2013)	• This philosophy is relatively new to the discussion of foundations for mixed methods research. • When used as the foundation for mixed methods, researchers tend to emphasize the importance of the context as part of the causation process, include both behavioral and mental phenomena in the research, and attend to diversity in individual meanings and contextual influences. • Critics of this foundation for mixed methods research note that it tends to downplay the epistemological

(Continued)

Table 8.1 (Continued)

Philosophy	Brief Description of the Ontological, Epistemological, and Axiological Assumptions[1]	Selected Mixed Methods Writings	Comments
			differences between the quantitative and qualitative approaches.
Postmodernism	• Reality is chaotic and unstructured. • All forms of knowledge are equal, and social structures are best examined through associated texts and discourse. • A researcher's values are an essential part of research but no better than others' values.	• Fielding (2008) • Freshwater (2007) • Hesse-Biber (2010b)	• This philosophy can be a foundation for mixed methods research, including critiquing unexamined aspects of mixed methods research practice and the field. • When used as the foundation for mixed methods, researchers tend to emphasize the use of mixed methods to challenge existing discourses in order to reveal inconsistencies within accepted practices and to stimulate new ways of thinking. • Critics of this foundation for mixed methods research note that it tends to reject many structures established within the field without offering meaningful alternatives.

[1]SOURCES: Christ (2013); Greene (2007); Hesse-Biber (2010b); Maxwell and Mittapalli (2010); Mertens (2003); Neuman (2011); Shannon-Baker (2015); Teddlie and Tashakkori (2009).

mixed methods research process) and the influences on those elements (i.e., mixed methods research content considerations and contexts). This theoretical model directly influenced how we have conceptualized and written about mixed methods research. For example, based on the configuration of this model, we waited to introduce the topic of "personal contexts" until late in the book, after first discussing the mixed methods research process and content considerations. In contrast, the authors of several other books about mixed methods research discussed the topic of personal contexts in the beginning chapter(s) (Creswell & Plano Clark, 2011; Greene, 2007; Hesse-Biber, 2010b; Teddlie & Tashakkori, 2009). In these other books, the authors approached mixed methods research using a theoretical model based on the stages of the research process, which placed personal contexts as the starting point for the research process.

As with all other forms of research, the use of theoretical models is important and common when researchers conduct mixed methods research studies (Creswell, 2015; Creswell, Klassen, Plano Clark, & Smith for the Office of Behavioral and Social Sciences Research, 2011). Scholars discuss the use of theory as a foundational component to mixed methods research in all of the prominent books in the field. These scholars tend to emphasize the critical role of theoretical models (along with philosophical assumptions) for determining research questions that call for a mixed methods approach (e.g., Creswell & Plano Clark, 2011; Hesse-Biber, 2010b; Teddlie & Tashakkori, 2009). Scholars also note that mixed methods researchers make different use of theory in their mixed methods studies. Three examples of ways to use theory in mixed methods research include using theory as an overarching stance for approaching the topic, deductively testing theory, and inductively generating theory. As introduced in Chapter 4, several rationales for using mixed methods relate to these different uses of theory (Bryman, 2006a). Morse and Niehaus (2009) went further by giving primary emphasis to the role of theory in mixed methods studies for classifying mixed methods designs. As noted in Chapter 5, they introduced the term *theoretical drive* to describe this role and argued that to be effective, mixed methods studies need to have a clear deductive theoretical drive (resulting in a quantitatively driven design) or inductive theoretical drive (resulting in a qualitatively driven design).

Whereas it is relatively easy to list the prominent philosophies discussed in the field of mixed methods research (see Table 8.1), it is impossible to capture even a meaningful subset of the social and behavioral theories that have been used in mixed methods research. Many theories are discipline specific and are generally used to guide research in their respective fields—for example, health belief model (in health behavior), social development theory (in education), and organizational theory (in business). One useful approach for thinking about the theoretical models used in mixed methods research is to consider the different types of theories that are found in mixed methods research practice, such as grand theories and middle-range theories (Ayres, 2008; Brewer, 2003). *Grand theories* (also referred to as *meta-theories* or *conceptual frameworks*) are highly abstract and untestable descriptions that provide an overall explanation of an organization to a discipline or body of knowledge. Examples of grand theories include socio-ecological theory, positive psychology, Marxist theory, and feminist theory. Within the field of mixed methods, grand theories are discussed in terms of providing a theoretical framework that guides all aspects of mixed methods research practice (recall the discussion of how scholars can intersect mixed methods research with a theoretical framework in Chapter 6). For example, Chen (2006) described the use of program theory as a conceptual framework that can guide the use of mixed methods research in evaluation.

In contrast to grand theories, *middle-range theories* are more focused and serve to describe the relationships among concepts for a particular phenomenon and suggest propositions that can be empirically tested. Examples of middle-range theories include diffusion of innovations theory, health behavior change theory, and motivation expectancy theory. When using mixed methods, researchers make many decisions based on their choice to use a middle-range theory such as to identify hypotheses, develop topic codes, and align quantitative and qualitative results to facilitate integration. For example, Brady and O'Regan (2009) described how they used Rhodes's theory of mentoring to design and integrate the quantitative and qualitative strands of their mixed methods study about the impacts of a youth mentoring program in Ireland.

Background Knowledge

Scholars' approaches to mixed methods research are also informed by their background knowledge. By **background knowledge,** we mean personal and professional experiences and expertise, including substantive and methodological training and skills, that provide the experiential foundation for a mixed methods research study. Each of us has amassed dispositions, preferences, and a lifetime of experiences that shape who we are as individuals but also who we are as researchers. This background can play an important role in one's research endeavors, including the use of mixed methods research. For example, practitioners who utilize quantitative and qualitative information in their professional practices (e.g., a family doctor who makes clinical decisions based on quantitative test results and a patient's descriptions) may be drawn to mixed methods research because it aligns well with their professional background. Similarly, researchers who have extensive expertise and experience with a particular research approach (e.g., randomized clinical trials) may be more likely to consider using mixed methods in ways that intersect with that approach (e.g., embedding a small qualitative component within a randomized clinical trial).

The role for background knowledge in mixed methods research is not always clear. Quantitative research traditions tend to value researchers' expertise for determining research questions, but also tend to be concerned with the potential for scholars' background knowledge to introduce bias into the research. Therefore, there is a tendency to use procedures to minimize this bias in quantitative research. In contrast, qualitative research traditions tend to value researchers' background knowledge, considering it as an essential guide for researchers' interpretations during the research process. Therefore, there is a tendency to use procedures that enhance the researchers' reflexivity about the role of their background in qualitative research. Not surprisingly, mixed methods research includes these two extreme perspectives along with all points between them. The mixed methods literature often acknowledges that researchers' background knowledge is important and influences mixed methods research practice (e.g., Greene, 2007; Hesse-Biber, 2010b; Teddlie & Tashakkori, 2009). Despite the importance of its role, it is not typical for researchers to formally discuss background knowledge in research reports. However, when mixed methods researchers are interviewed about their mixed methods research practices, they highlight the importance of their personal background knowledge for thinking about and applying mixed methods research (Bryman, 2006b, 2007; Leech, 2010; Plano Clark, 2005). One related topic that is receiving extensive attention in the mixed methods literature at this time is the role of researchers' methodological training and skills in mixed methods research. The literature notes the importance of training for shaping researchers' mixed methods research practices and discusses the wide array of personal dispositions and qualitative, quantitative, and mixed methods skill sets required to implement rigorous mixed methods studies (Brannen, 2005; Creswell, 2015; Curry & Nunez-Smith, 2015; Morgan, 2014).

STANCES ABOUT PERSONAL
CONTEXTS FOR MIXED METHODS RESEARCH

Unquestionably, scholars' philosophical assumptions, theoretical models, and background knowledge are dynamically interrelated to form their personal contexts for mixed methods research. Greene (2007), in particular, has drawn attention to this issue in the field by discussing the role of *mental models* in mixed methods research. She defined mental models as "the particular constellation of assumptions, theoretical commitments, experiences, and values through which a social inquirer conducts his or her work" (p. 3). She discussed how our mental models—made up of our assumptions, theories, and experiences—not only provide the lens for using mixed methods research but also are at the core of what it means to mix methods. That is, her stance suggests that the very nature of mixed methods research is to bring multiple mental models into conversation within the study of a particular phenomenon.

Although all three aspects of personal contexts are addressed in the mixed methods literature, none has received as extensive attention as researchers' philosophical assumptions, and philosophical foundations are often described as being intertwined with scholars' theoretical models and background knowledge. The implications of researchers' philosophical assumptions for mixed methods research has been a prominent and hotly debated topic in the mixed methods literature. As part of these discussions, scholars have actively compared the different philosophies as providing foundations for mixed methods (e.g., Greene, 2007; Johnson & Onwuegbuzie, 2004; Teddlie & Tashakkori, 2009), debated the multiple meanings of philosophies and paradigms and their role in the field (e.g., Freshwater & Cahill, 2013; Morgan, 2007), considered the relative prevalence of certain philosophies (e.g., Alise & Teddlie, 2010; Giddings & Grant, 2007), and discussed the implications of different philosophical stances for the conduct of mixed methods research (e.g., Christ, 2013; Greene & Hall, 2010; Shannon-Baker, 2015).

Among all of these writings, several stances exist regarding the connections between philosophical assumptions and mixed methods research (Creswell & Plano Clark, 2011; Greene, 2007; Teddlie & Tashakkori, 2009). The stances represent different perspectives about the meaning and importance of research philosophies for mixed methods research practice. One prominent stance is that *one* set of philosophical assumptions can provide a good foundation for mixed methods research. Looking back at Table 8.1, you should note that pragmatism, critical realism, and the transformative–emancipatory perspective are each identified by scholars as a philosophy that researchers can adopt and use to inform and shape their decisions about mixed methods research content and mixed methods research practice. For example, Curry and Nunez-Smith (2015) noted how their approach to mixed methods research, as described in their book for health sciences researchers, is shaped by their self-identification as pragmatists. As they summed up, "We consider ourselves to be pragmatists. . . . Simply put, we use whatever works" (p. xxii). This using-what-works approach is found throughout their book as they focus on very practical strategies and designs for researchers to apply in their own mixed methods research practice.

Another prominent stance within the mixed methods literature is to argue for the use of an overarching perspective that guides the use of multiple, even conflicting, sets of philosophical assumptions within mixed methods studies. Returning to Table 8.1, you should note that the dialectical perspective and dialectical pluralism are explicit frameworks that support using two or more sets of assumptions within one mixed methods study. For example, Onwuegbuzie, Rosli, Ingram, and Frels (2014) combined a critical, social justice stance with phenomenological assumptions and postpositivist assumptions in their transformative, sequential mixed research study of the experiences of women doctoral students. In their study report, they clearly articulated how different philosophical assumptions provided the foundation for different study components as well as the integration of the different components in the analysis. They noted that their procedures were "consistent with our critical dialectical pluralist stance" (p. 10).

ISSUES AND DEBATES ABOUT PERSONAL CONTEXTS AND MIXED METHODS RESEARCH

Considering the many different perspectives that exist about mixed methods research, it should come as no surprise that personal contexts remain one of the most discussed and controversial issues in the field of mixed methods research. Here, we briefly introduce four issues that continue to be discussed and debated within the field.

1. Can you really mix and integrate research philosophies (or methods)? An important debate for mixed methods research is whether philosophies (and their associated methods) can logically be mixed. We have already introduced two stances for responding to this question: (1) There are single philosophies that can provide a strong foundation for mixing methods and therefore do not require philosophies to be mixed, and (2) a dialectical perspective can provide a strong foundation for thoughtfully combining two or more philosophies. These two stances represent many scholars in the field of mixed methods research. However, for others who are referred to as "purists," the answer to whether different philosophies and methods can be mixed is "no, they cannot." The history of the field of mixed methods research took root in the quantitative–qualitative debate (also referred to as the *paradigm wars*) that occupied research communities in the second half of the twentieth century (Tashakkori & Teddlie, 1998). As scholars across disciplines more clearly differentiated philosophies (e.g., postpositivism and constructivism) and considered their implications for research practice, many reached the conclusion that different philosophies cannot be logically mixed and integrated. That is, some scholars have concluded that researchers *cannot* assume that there is a single reality independent from the researcher while also assuming that multiple constructed realities exist because those two beliefs are inherently illogical when combined. From this perspective, several have argued that mixed methods research is untenable because you cannot mix methods that are based in incompatible views of the social world (e.g., Sale, Lohfeld, & Brazil, 2002; Smith, 1983). Although this is not a predominant view currently, it highlights one reason why you need to thoughtfully consider the stance and assumptions that form the foundation for your mixed methods research practice and be prepared to respond to others' concerns that mixed methods research is fundamentally illogical.

2. Must you align with one formal research philosophy? There are actually many different views about research philosophies, their relationship to individuals, and their role in research practice. A significant component of these ongoing debates is the many definitions of paradigms found in the literature (Freshwater & Cahill, 2013). Although much of the literature discusses philosophical assumptions in terms of formal research philosophies (as we did in Table 8.1), that is not the only perspective. For example, some have noted that such views are socially constructed and agreed upon by groups, such as research communities or disciplines; therefore, other authors focus less on the assumptions held by individuals (e.g., Denscombe, 2008). (We will discuss disciplinary contexts for mixed methods research in Chapter 10.) As another example, Maxwell (2011) argued that individuals should adopt an approach he referred to as *bricolage* by viewing philosophical positions as practical tools and carefully assembling a toolkit of assumptions and perspectives that most usefully fit the researchers' personal contexts and particular research situation. Although many (perhaps countless) perspectives exist regarding individuals' philosophical assumptions for mixed methods, scholars generally agree that the most important aspect is for you to both consider and clearly articulate the assumptions that inform your use of mixed methods research and how they shape its use.

3. How best to incorporate theoretical models into mixed methods research? Although there are many different perspectives on most topics in the mixed methods literature, it appears that all authors agree that the use of theory is important for mixed methods research practice (e.g., Creswell et al., 2011). The issue that is starting to receive more attention, however, is *how* scholars can meaningfully incorporate theory into their mixed methods research practices and report their use of theory in their mixed methods reports (Creswell, 2015; Evans Coon, & Ume, 2011). Some authors have discussed the use of certain theories (e.g., substantive or social justice) in con-nection with specific mixed methods designs (e.g., Creswell & Plano Clark, 2011; Mertens, 2003; Teddlie & Tashakkori, 2009), but different types of theories may be used and incorporated at different levels (e.g., used as an overarching theoretical framework or used in only one of the strands). To date, there is relatively little guidance on the different uses of theory in mixed methods research compared to the guidance found in the discussions of quan-titative and qualitative research traditions. Despite the lack of guidance, you should attend to the use of theory within your own and others' mixed methods research practices.

4. What training is needed to conduct mixed methods research? The issue of training and skills for mixed methods research is another topic of growing concern and interest (Creswell, 2015; Creswell et al., 2011). Although there are several discussions in the literature regarding the training and skills needed in mixed methods research teams (a topic we will discuss in Chapter 9), how to best address this information for individual researchers is still unset-tled. What are the minimum competencies that you need in terms of quantita-tive research training and skills and qualitative research training and skills?

What training and skills do you need in terms of mixed methods research? How do you obtain these advanced skills if you are an emerging scholar just learning to conduct research? How do you obtain these specialized skills to augment your research training if you are a senior scholar who is well into your career? You need to find the answers to these questions within your own research contexts to develop the necessary expertise to be able to implement rigorous, high-quality mixed methods research practices.

These four questions highlight some of the ongoing debates and lingering issues in the field about personal contexts for mixed methods research. They also point to the importance placed on scholars explicitly articulating their personal assumptions and experiences that provide the contexts for their mixed methods research practices. These differing opinions acknowledge that each of us brings our own viewpoints and experiences to the field of mixed methods research and that the field is broad and inclusive enough to welcome us all.

APPLYING PERSONAL CONTEXTS IN MIXED METHODS RESEARCH PRACTICE

As we have discussed throughout this chapter, your mixed methods research practices are shaped by who you are as a researcher and your philosophical assumptions, theoretical models, and background knowledge. The field of mixed methods research ascribes significant importance to these personal contexts for all scholars who apply mixed methods research because of the influential role they play in mixed methods research content considerations and the research process. Although the perspectives about personal contexts are about as diverse as the number of scholars who engage in mixed methods research practices, collectively authors writing in the field have advanced the expectation that researchers both thoughtfully consider and fully acknowledge their role in all forms of mixed methods research practice including reading about, applying, evaluating, or teaching mixed methods research. In Box 8.1, we offer some general advice for applying the concepts of this chapter to your mixed methods research practice.

When reading and reviewing the literature about mixed methods research, it is critical to consider the authors' philosophical assumptions, theoretical models, and background knowledge because they have important influences

---

Box 8.1

Advice for Applying Personal Contexts in Mixed Methods Research Practice

Advice for Reading/Reviewing Mixed Methods Studies and Methodological Discussions

- Recognize that all scholars who engage in mixed methods research practices come with their own personal contexts (i.e., philosophical assumptions, theoretical models, and background knowledge).
- Remember that many differences exist among scholars' personal contexts, which have important implications for their mixed methods research practices.
- Look for statements written by the author that explicitly identified the philosophical assumptions, theoretical models, and background knowledge that shaped her or his mixed methods research practice. If not stated explicitly, look for clues in how the author considered mixed methods research content and made decisions about a study's research process.
- Assess the extent to which the author has clearly articulated (and supported by citations to the literature) her or his philosophical assumptions, theoretical models, and background knowledge as foundations for the mixed methods research practice.
- Assess the extent to which the author's mixed methods research practice was consistent with her or his philosophical assumptions, theoretical models, and background knowledge.

Advice for Proposing/Reporting/Discussing Mixed Methods Research

- Reflect on your philosophical assumptions, theoretical models, and background knowledge and how these personal contexts provide the foundation for your mixed methods research practice.
- Identify formal philosophies and theories discussed in the literature that align with your personal philosophical assumptions and theoretical models.
- Explicitly identify the personal contexts that inform your mixed methods research practice, and support those positions with citations from the scholarly literature.

(Continued)

(Continued)

- Explain how and why your personal contexts shape your perspectives about the mixed methods research content considerations and your decisions about the mixed methods research process.
- Ensure that your mixed methods research practice is aligned with your philosophical assumptions, theoretical models, and background knowledge.

on how mixed methods research is applied. It is useful to remember that there is great diversity in the personal contexts of the scholars who are part of the field of mixed methods research (Harrits, 2011). This diversity leads to many different perspectives about mixed methods research content considerations and different decisions for the mixed methods research process. By identifying the philosophical assumptions, theoretical models, and background knowledge of the author(s), you will be well positioned to both understand and assess the quality of the mixed methods research practice. Keep in mind that there is no one "right" set of contexts for mixed methods research. However, scholars do need to discuss and apply mixed methods research in ways that are logically consistent with their philosophical, theoretical, and experiential foundations.

It is also critically important to reflect on your own personal contexts when you design and report your own mixed methods study. Your philosophical assumptions, theoretical models, and background knowledge are part of your mixed methods research efforts and play a role in your decisions from how you define mixed methods, to how you consider quality, to how you integrate and draw inferences from your quantitative and qualitative results. If left unexamined, your personal contexts may lead to problematic biases and illogical mixed methods research practices. However, when you carefully examine and clearly explain your personal contexts, they provide a solid foundation from which to base your applications of mixed methods research. Although the extent to which you explicitly discuss your philosophical assumptions, theoretical models, and background knowledge within a proposal or report may be influenced by reviewers' expectations (a topic to be further discussed in Chapter 9), you will still find that your use of mixed methods research will benefit from clearly identifying your foundations, supporting them with relevant literature, and using them to guide your mixed methods research practice.

CONCLUDING COMMENTS

We conclude the chapter by offering some final summary comments organized by the learning objectives stated at the beginning of the chapter.

- **Understand different personal contexts for mixed methods research.** Scholars approach their use of mixed methods research from their own personal contexts. These personal contexts include philosophical assumptions about reality and how knowledge about reality can be gained, theoretical models about the nature of the topic being studied, and background knowledge including personal and professional experience and training.
- **Recognize how philosophical assumptions, theoretical models, and background knowledge provide foundations for mixed methods research practice.** Philosophical assumptions, theoretical models, and background knowledge directly influence mixed methods research practice. These personal contexts shape scholars' perspectives about mixed methods content considerations, including how it is defined, why it is used, what designs are considered, how it is intersected with other approaches, and how quality is assessed. In addition, these personal contexts also influence researchers' decisions about the research process such as the research questions that are posed; the timing, integration, and priority of the methods; and the inferences that are drawn.
- **Describe different stances about personal contexts for mixed methods research.** A prominent stance in mixed methods research is that the assumptions from one research philosophy (e.g., pragmatism, critical realism, or the transformative–emancipatory perspective) can provide a strong foundation for mixed methods research. In contrast, a dialectical or pluralistic stance argues that a strong foundation for mixed methods research is to incorporate a thoughtful dialogue between two or more sets of philosophical assumptions (e.g., postpositivism and constructivism). A contrasting historical stance is the viewpoint that philosophies—and therefore methods—cannot be logically mixed and therefore rigorous mixed methods research is not possible.

APPLICATION QUESTIONS

1. Locate a published mixed methods research study from your area of interest and, based on the information included in the article, identify the researchers' personal contexts that provided the foundations for the study in the form of philosophical assumptions, theoretical models, and background knowledge.

2. Locate two articles (methodological discussions or empirical studies) about mixed methods research that are each aligned with a different philosophical stance for mixed methods research. Make a list of the differences you note in how the authors discussed and applied mixed methods research, and discuss how those differences align with the different personal contexts of the authors.

3. Consider your own personal contexts and list examples of the philosophical assumptions, theoretical models, and background knowledge that you bring to your area of interest and use of mixed methods research. Describe how these personal contexts might directly influence your mixed methods research practice.

4. Pick one of the ongoing issues and debates about personal contexts for mixed methods research: whether philosophies can be mixed in research, whether researchers must align with a formal philosophy, the lack of guidance for using theory in mixed methods research, and the training required to conduct mixed methods research. State why you selected that issue, and discuss your reactions to this issue in terms of foundations for the use of mixed methods research.

KEY RESOURCES

To learn more about personal contexts for mixed methods research, we suggest you start with the following resources:

1. **Teddlie, C., & Tashakkori, A. (2009). Paradigm issues in mixed methods research. In** *Foundations of mixed methods research: Integrating quantitative and qualitative approaches in the social and behavioral sciences* **(pp. 83–105). Thousand Oaks, CA: Sage.**

   • In this chapter, Teddlie and Tashakkori provided a historical overview of the different major philosophies that are discussed in the field of mixed methods research along with debates that have occurred over time.

*2. **Morgan, D. L. (2007). Paradigms lost and pragmatism regained: Methodological implications of combining qualitative and quantitative methods.** *Journal of Mixed Methods Research, 1*(1), 48–76.

- In this article, Morgan provided an in-depth discussion of the evolving importance of philosophical issues for research communities, with a specific focus on the tenets of pragmatism and how they provide a foundation for mixed methods research.

3. **Greene, J. C., & Hall, J. N. (2010). Dialectics and pragmatism: Being of consequence. In A. Tashakkori & C. Teddlie (Eds.),** *SAGE handbook of mixed methods in social & behavioral research* **(2nd ed., pp. 119–143). Thousand Oaks, CA: Sage.**

- In this chapter, Greene and Hall provided a practical discussion about the differences between using one set of philosophical assumptions (i.e., pragmatism) and using a dialectic of two sets of philosophical assumptions, including the implications of these differences for two examples of mixed methods research practice.

*4. **Mertens, D. M. (2007). Transformative paradigm: Mixed methods and social justice.** *Journal of Mixed Methods Research, 1*(3), 212–225.

- In this article, Mertens discussed the role of philosophical assumptions in mixed methods research and articulated the assumptions and practices associated with a transformative–emancipatory perspective and social justice theories.

5. **Creswell, J. W. (2015). Skills needed to conduct mixed methods research. In J. W. Creswell,** *A concise introduction to mixed methods research* **(pp. 23–33). Thousand Oaks, CA: Sage.**

- In this chapter, Creswell discussed the training and skills needed to provide researchers with a strong foundation for conducting mixed methods research.

* The key resource is available at the following website: http://study.sagepub.com/planoclark.

NINE

HOW DO INTERPERSONAL CONTEXTS SHAPE MIXED METHODS?

CONSIDERING INTERACTIONS WITH RESEARCH PARTICIPANTS, TEAMS, AND REVIEWERS IN MIXED METHODS RESEARCH

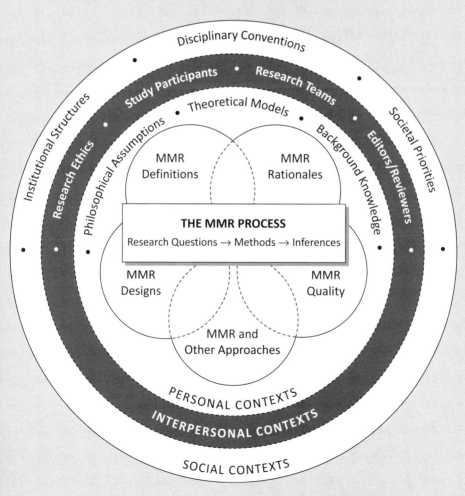

*N*ow that you understand the role of personal contexts in influencing researchers' approaches to the practice of mixed methods research, it is important to think about the influences of the interpersonal contexts that form the next level in our socio-ecological framework for mixed methods research. These contexts include considerations of research ethics, complex relationships with research participants, evolving dynamics of research teams, and compliance with editorial and review boards of the journals that publish mixed methods research. In this chapter, we describe these relationships, introduce perspectives and debates related to interpersonal contexts, and offer recommendations for how to understand and address interpersonal contexts in mixed methods research practice.

LEARNING OBJECTIVES

This chapter aims to provide you with an understanding of interpersonal contexts that shape mixed methods research content considerations and the research process so you are able to do the following:

- Understand different interpersonal contexts for mixed methods research.
- Recognize how considerations related to compliance with research ethics, research participants, research team dynamics, and relationships with editorial and review boards shape mixed methods research practice.
- Describe practical approaches for addressing interpersonal contexts for mixed methods research.

CHAPTER 9 KEY CONCEPTS

The following key concepts will help you navigate through the main considerations related to interpersonal contexts for mixed methods research as they are introduced in this chapter:

- **Interpersonal contexts:** Research ethics and researchers' relationships with study participants, research teams, and editorial and review boards that shape mixed methods research practice.

- **Mixed methods research ethics:** A set of moral principles that are aimed at assisting researchers in conducting mixed methods research ethically and in compliance with existing standards for research involving humans.
- **Research participant considerations:** Issues that researchers have to address when engaging participants in research; these issues may relate to gaining access and recruiting study participants, involving community members as research partners, studying vulnerable populations, and considering cultural contexts that shape participants' experiences.
- **Research team dynamics:** Relationships and interactions among the members of a research team that influence their approaches to the mixed methods research process used in a study.
- **Editorial and review board guidelines:** Criteria established by journal editorial boards for authors to follow when submitting manuscripts for publishing consideration and by which their work will be appraised and judged.

THE ROLE OF INTERPERSONAL CONTEXTS IN THE FIELD OF MIXED METHODS RESEARCH

As we described in Chapter 8, researchers' philosophical assumptions, theoretical orientation, and background knowledge influence their approaches to designing and conducting a mixed methods study and shape their decisions about what methods to employ and emphasize during the mixed methods research process. However, knowledge generation is a collaborative process and requires collegial interactions among many stakeholders that influence how the study is designed, implemented, and reported (McNiff & Whitehead, 2011). As researchers conceptualize and conduct their mixed methods studies, they enter a complex system of relationships with study participants, co-researchers, and other audiences. These "outside factors" play an important role because they create the power dynamics that influence the mixed methods research process used in a study (Morgan, 2014, p. 232). For example, as a researcher, you must adhere to ethical norms and principles for research with humans and consider how to address the needs of different study populations when engaging them in research. Since most of mixed methods research is done in teams, you have to take into account the changing dynamics of collaborating with other investigators, project advisory boards, and participant co-researchers. In addition, when you report your mixed methods study or review research done by others, you have to keep in mind how your work will be accepted and evaluated by different audiences, including other scholars, your academic advisors and dissertation committee members, journal reviewers, policy makers, and the lay public.

We define this system of relationships as **interpersonal contexts,** which include research ethics and researchers' relationships with study participants, research teams, and editorial and review boards that shape the practice of mixed methods research. As shown in Figure 9.1, interpersonal contexts form another layer in our socio-ecological framework for mixed methods research and influence researchers' personal contexts in how they apply their beliefs

Figure 9.1 The Role of Interpersonal Contexts in the Practice of Mixed Methods Research

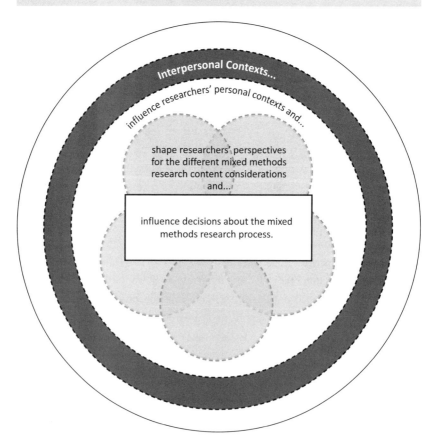

and background knowledge when engaging in mixed methods research. Likewise, through personal contexts, interpersonal contexts shape researchers' perspectives for each mixed methods research content domain that, in turn, influence and shape the decisions researchers make about the mixed methods research process. Therefore, understanding the role of interpersonal contexts along with other contexts and methodological domains is important for you to successfully navigate the field of mixed methods research.

MAJOR PERSPECTIVES ABOUT INTERPERSONAL CONTEXTS FOR MIXED METHODS RESEARCH

Interpersonal contexts constitute an integral dimension of any interpersonal interactions that involve exchange of information (Holtgraves, 1992), which also includes the process of research. While considering interpersonal contexts is important in any type of research, the role of interpersonal contexts has received more attention in the qualitative research literature due to the interactive and interpersonal nature of this form of inquiry (e.g., Hemmings, 2005; Hesse-Biber & Leavy, 2011; Hewitt, 2007; Morse, 2007; Padgett, 2012). In the mixed methods research field, the issues of interpersonal contexts are gaining more interest as the popularity of mixed methods is growing and expanding across disciplines. The process and the outcomes of mixed methods research is oftentimes a joint group endeavor that is marked by different tangible values, interdisciplinary traditions, and cultural norms (Johnson, Onwuegbuzie, Tucker, & Icenogle, 2014). A body of literature is emerging in the field of mixed methods research that addresses the interpersonal contexts of conducting mixed methods research, although these issues are often embedded in the larger discussions of mixed methods theory and practice. To help you understand these influences, we discuss the emergent perspectives on interpersonal contexts organized as four broad, often-interrelated categories: mixed methods research ethics, research participant considerations, research team dynamics, and editorial and review board guidelines.

Mixed Methods Research Ethics

Conducting research with humans necessitates compliance with ethical standards aimed at protecting study participants from the risk of harmful effects and ensuring their well-being (National Commission for the Protection of Human Subjects, 1979). As you engage in mixed methods research, you must comply with the principles of **mixed methods research ethics,** which we define as a set of moral principles that are aimed at assisting researchers in conducting mixed methods research ethically and in compliance with existing standards for research involving humans. Therefore, before a study inception, researchers are required to seek its approval from a local ethical review board, which sometimes may be time consuming due to a sensitive study topic and require several iterations to satisfy the board requirements. In addition, researchers need to solicit an informed consent from each study participant, disclose the study procedures, ensure participants' confidentiality, and abide by appropriate codes of professional conduct. Many national and international professional organizations have codes of research ethics that, in addition to general principles of research ethics, address ethical standards of conducting research specific for each field.

Although the same general principles of research ethics apply in mixed methods research (Teddlie & Tashakkori, 2009), the logistics of the mixed methods research process call for additional ethical considerations (Brewer & Hunter, 1989). These issues are discussed in the emergent literature on mixed methods research ethics (Curry & Nunez-Smith, 2015; Hesse-Biber, 2010b; Ivankova, 2015; Plowright, 2011; Preissle, Glover-Kudon, Rohan, Boehm, & DeGroff, 2015; Teddlie & Tashakkori, 2009). Teddlie and Tashakkori (2009) warranted that it is important to consider the context and demands of both quantitative and qualitative research procedures and settings within one ethical review board application. Because collecting quantitative and qualitative data entails different levels of data sensitivity—for example, using standardized instruments versus unstructured open-ended interview guides—an ethical review board may require explanations of different details related to these processes. Hesse-Biber (2010b) discussed ethical dilemmas specific to different stages of a mixed methods study and offered insights into the complexity of the informed consent due to the need to link responses to study participants in sequential designs. Ethical concerns increase in advanced applications of mixed methods designs when researchers intersect mixed methods with other research methodologies due to their methodological specificity. For example, in mixed methods action research, three sets of ethical issues must be considered: responsible conduct of research in general; issues of power, ownership, and participation in action research; and limited anonymity and demands of time commitment for participants in mixed methods research (Ivankova, 2015).

Plowright (2011) provided a thorough discussion of the ethical issues that mixed methods researchers should be prepared to expect when working with study participants due to influences of numerous professional, organizational, and policy contexts. Likewise, the growing interest in mixed methods research in the health sciences promoted a detailed discussion of the ethical issues for researchers to consider when developing a mixed methods research proposal for National Institutes of Health (NIH) funding (Creswell, Klassen, Plano Clark, & Smith for the Office of Behavioral and Social Sciences Research, 2011; Curry & Nunez-Smith, 2015). These emergent discussions underscore the complexity of the ethical issues researchers face in their mixed methods research practice and call for a continued dialogue on this important topic.

Research Participant Considerations

Research ethics has a direct relationship to how you approach and address the needs of research participants when you involve them in mixed methods projects. **Research participant considerations** form another important aspect of interpersonal contexts to address and include issues related to gaining access and recruiting study participants, involving community members as research partners, studying vulnerable populations, and considering cultural contexts that shape participants' experiences. In addition to the issues of recruiting and retaining study participants that are common to quantitative and qualitative research, designing and conducting a mixed methods study pose challenges associated with increased time commitment from participants necessary for collecting both types of data, the need to obtain participants' identifying information for follow-up purposes, and the potential loss of participants for follow-up in sequential designs (Creswell et al., 2011; Curry & Nunez-Smith, 2015; Morse & Niehaus, 2009). Additional challenges arise when researchers need to combine mixed methods with participatory and community-based research approaches or aim to study vulnerable populations.

Engaging study participants as co-researchers and active partners in the research process challenges researchers' capacity to learn through collaboration and to construct joint meanings of the data. At the same time, an increased interest in participatory approaches to research and focus on patient-centered outcomes (Curry, Nembhard, & Bradley, 2009; Ivankova, 2015; Olson & Jason, 2015) have provided a platform for engaging stakeholders with mixed methods research projects (see also the discussion about intersecting mixed methods with action research in Chapter 6). Shulha and Wilson (2003) referred to mixed methods research as being collaborative in nature because it offers "the purposeful application of a multiple person, multiple perspective approach to questions of research and evaluation" (p. 640). Community-based participatory research (CBPR) provides a viable venue for expanding mixed methods research to communities and soliciting "the active engagement and influence of community members in all aspects of the research process" (Israel, Schulz, Parker, & Becker, 2001, p. 184). Combining mixed methods with a CBPR approach is particularly effective in developing culturally tailored interventions by facilitating the inclusion of community perspectives in all phases of the research process (Nastasi, Hitchcock, & Brown, 2010; Nastasi & Hitchcock, 2016; Windsor, 2013). Eisinger and Senturia (2001) suggested that participation, equal power, and joint planning are three key principles that form the foundation of CBPR. You should consider these principles when establishing collaborative relationships with community partners and developing mixed methods research strategies aimed at community well-being.

Important considerations should also be given to using mixed methods to study vulnerable and marginalized groups. These considerations relate to gaining access to special populations, involving them as research participants, establishing trust relationships, preserving their perspectives and values, and adopting an advocacy and social justice perspective. There is a growing body of the mixed methods literature that focuses on these issues. A recent special issue of the *Journal of Mixed Methods Research* (JMMR) provides a discussion of engaging the underserved and vulnerable populations in research using a transformative mixed methods approach (Marti & Mertens, 2014). The collection of articles written by international authors provides insight into using mixed methods research with different vulnerable groups, such as individuals with spinal cord injuries (Sullivan, Derrett, Paul, Beaver, & Stace, 2014); deaf people (Wilson & Winiarczyk, 2014); students from disadvantaged economic backgrounds (Shuayb, 2014); vulnerable children from developing countries (Kim, 2014); ethnic and indigenous communities (Chilisa & Tsheko, 2014); and lesbian, gay, bisexual, and transgender groups (Zea, Aguilar-Pardo, Betancourt, Reisen, & Gonzales, 2014). In addition, there are numerous publications that illustrate effective mixed methods strategies to studying marginalized groups, such as combining mixed methods with participatory and action research approaches, policy analysis, concept mapping, analysis of existing databases, and epidemiological designs. We present a few select examples from different disciplines along with our comments related to the use of mixed methods to address the issue in Table 9.1. We suggest you explore these examples and comments to better understand how mixed methods can facilitate research with vulnerable populations to help address the issues of social and health disparities (see also the discussion about intersecting mixed methods with theoretical frameworks in Chapter 6).

Research Team Dynamics

The breadth and scope of mixed methods research often requires expertise in multiple research methods and content areas, which calls for a collaborative team approach. The dynamics of research teams creates another interpersonal context to consider when you engage in mixed methods research practice. We define *research team dynamics* as relationships and interactions among the members of a research team that influence their approaches to the mixed methods research process. Mixed methods research teams often include researchers from different disciplines and methodological traditions, who combine their knowledge and expertise to work together on designing and implementing a study. Along with the necessary knowledge and research skills, they bring their personal, professional, organizational, and cultural identities that influence the team dynamics. While the diversity is welcome and encouraged in mixed methods teams, it can also provoke tensions within interdisciplinary research teams (Hemmings, Beckett, Kennerly, & Yap, 2013; O'Cathain, Murphy, & Nicholl, 2008) and create barriers to effective collaboration and achieving the study goals (Curry et al., 2012).

With the expansion of mixed methods research across disciplines, team dynamics has received increased attention in the mixed methods literature. Mixed methods authors have advanced different perspectives about how to understand and address the research team dynamics. Hemmings and colleagues (2013) discussed "discipline-bordered" social dynamics (p. 263) that occur in interdisciplinary mixed methods teams across education and nursing using "communities of practice" (Denscombe, 2008, p. 270) as a framework for understanding mixed methods research. Johnson and colleagues (2014) proposed the dialectical pluralism implementation framework as a philosophical foundation for constructing mixed methods teams and dealing with the group processes related to different values and perspectives of the team members. Several perspectives have been advanced to address mixed methods team dynamics in health sciences research. Curry and colleagues (2012) used the representational group theory of intergroup relations along with

Table 9.1 Select Examples of Using Mixed Methods Research to Study Vulnerable Groups

Publication	Discipline	Vulnerable Population	Issue Addressed	Mixed Methods Use	Comments
Craig (2011)	• Social work	• Lesbian, gay, bisexual, transgender, and questioning (LGBTQ) youths	• Assessing the needs of and developing a system of care for LGBTQ youths in an urban area	• Mixed methods combined with community-based participatory research (CBPR) and action research	• Focus on the strategies of involvement of community and LGBTQ youths, using mixed methods for problem and needs assessment.
Windsor (2013)	• Health	• Alcohol and substance users	• Health disparities in predominantly African American and distressed communities	• Mixed methods combined with CBPR and concept mapping	• Focus on the advantages of combining mixed methods with CBPR and concept mapping for developing culturally tailored and community-based health interventions for vulnerable populations.

Shepard, Orsi, Mahon, and Carroll (2002)	• Nursing	• Vulnerable families (including a member with HIV/ AIDS or other life-threatening conditions, or a child with a chronic condition)	• Complex reality of living as a vulnerable family	• Mixed methods combined with prospective cohort study and longitudinal approaches	• Focus on advancing mixed methods as a research approach to studying vulnerable families in nursing science.
Kohrt (2009)	• Psychology	• Vulnerable social groups based on caste and ethnicity	• Psychosocial morbidity and caste issues among vulnerable social groups in post conflict settings in Nepal	• Mixed methods combined with policy analysis and epidemiology	• Focus on using mixed methods as a framework for designing and implementing psychosocial intervention programs in post conflict settings.
Chankseliani (2013)	• Education	• Young college applicants from economically disadvantaged rural areas	• Disparities in admission to Georgian higher education institutions for rural applicants	• Mixed methods combined with a secondary analysis of a national data set and individual in-depth interviews	• Focus on the advantages of mixed methods to integrate broad trends at the national level with details from an in-depth individual-level inquiry.

227

their personal experiences to explain the challenges that researchers face when working in teams on mixed methods projects in the health sciences. Their perspective emphasizes the dynamics that researchers bring into the project "*both* as individuals and as members of a variety of groups" (p. 7). Likewise, Creswell and colleagues (2011) used Rosenfield's (1992) taxonomy of three levels of collaborative research between social and health scientists (multidisciplinary, interdisciplinary, and transdisciplinary) to inform their discussion of the roles of research teams in developing successful NIH grant applications.

Editorial and Review Board Guidelines

When you report or review mixed methods research, you experience the influence of another type of interpersonal contexts—that is, you have to comply with **editorial and review board guidelines.** These are the criteria established by journal editorial boards for the authors to follow when submitting manuscripts for publishing consideration and by which their work will be appraised and judged. Most journals that publish research have editorial and review boards that consist of content experts and methodologists that review, evaluate, and make judgment about the quality of the submitted manuscripts. This process is referred to as *peer review* and is shaped by shared cultural and academic norms and standards existing in disciplines (Becher & Trowler, 2001). The guidelines for authors are often set in accordance with the epistemological traditions and scientific norms adopted in different disciplines emphasizing either a quantitative or a qualitative approach and also the levels of acceptance of mixed methods research within the disciplines (we will further discuss the influences of disciplinary conventions in Chapter 10). The allowed word limit for a manuscript length often imposes additional challenges for reporting a mixed methods study "in its entirety" (Cameron, 2011, p. 98). To comply with these guidelines, authors often have to put more emphasis on reporting the results from either a quantitative or a qualitative study strand or publish their mixed methods studies as separate quantitative and qualitative papers.

The emergent literature on the challenges of publishing mixed methods research underscores the importance of their influences on mixed methods research practice. Cameron (2011) discussed the political nature of publishing mixed methods research in academic and discipline-based literature and connected it to the views expressed by Tashakkori and Teddlie (2010a) that mixed methods along with qualitative research is still viewed as positioned "outside the mainstream in certain disciplines" (Cameron, 2011, p. 105). Additionally, the peer review process used by the journals was criticized for serving to rein-force the existing quality norms and methodological standards rather than establish the new criteria more acceptable of mixed methods (Hurtado, 2012; Papadimitriou, Ivankova, & Hurtado, 2013). Oftentimes, reviewers are trained in one method or have some familiarity with both quantitative and qualitative research, but only occasionally is a reviewer "well-versed in the most recent developments in mixed methods research" (Papadimitriou et al., 2013, p. 150). The challenges of the peer review process for mixed methods research have also been discussed in the recent works by Dahlberg, Wittink, and Gallo (2010) and Curry and Nunez-Smith (2015), such as accepting the criticism from those who may have little experience with mixed methods, deciding what reviewers' comments will strengthen the manuscript, preparing the revised manuscript, and developing a response letter to the editor explaining the ratio-nale for the changes and the reasons for using mixed methods.

Similar challenges are faced by master's and doctoral students as they prepare their mixed methods study proposals or completed reports for review by academic advisors and committee members. Graduate students using a mixed methods approach for their research projects often take on the addi-tional responsibility of needing to educate committee members about mixed methods and clearly explaining and justifying their procedures. Adding to the challenge is the fact that explicit guidelines for writing master's theses and dissertations rarely exist and students need to learn about the expectations that are specific to their program, committee members, and advisor. Understanding these and other challenges imposed by interpersonal contexts and learning how to address them will better position you to practice mixed methods research. In the following section, we provide some examples of addressing interpersonal contexts in practice drawn from the mixed methods literature.

EXAMPLES OF ADDRESSING INTERPERSONAL CONTEXTS IN MIXED METHODS RESEARCH PRACTICE

As we described previously, the influences of interpersonal contexts can sig-nificantly impact the mixed methods research process. Therefore, it is impor-tant to understand and find ways to successfully address these influences from engaging research participants in mixed methods studies, to learning how to work in mixed methods project teams, to educating others about mixed methods research. Despite the paucity of practical suggestions of how to deal with the influences of interpersonal contexts in mixed methods research, we provide the available recommendations for three types of contexts as they are addressed in the mixed methods literature: mixed methods research ethics, research team dynamics, and editorial and review board guidelines. We organize these recommendations in respective tables and provide our comments about each set of recommendations, consisting of the disciplinary contexts, the authors' methodological orientation, the guiding theoretical perspective, and the practical implications of these recommendations for mixed methods research practice.

We begin with the recommendations for addressing ethical issues in mixed methods studies. The mixed methods literature offers a few practical suggestions about how to deal with different ethical review board requirements for collecting quantitative and qualitative data within one study and also how to address ethical issues related to the sequential nature of some mixed methods designs (Hesse-Biber, 2010b). As we noted earlier, mixed methods research ethics has thus far received more attention among the health sciences researchers evidently due to the growing number of mixed methods funded studies. Creswell and colleagues (2011) developed a detailed outline of the procedures for the protection of human subjects in NIH research applications, whereas Curry and Nunez-Smith (2015) provided helpful tips for preparing a strong mixed methods research application for human research protection program review. We summarized and discussed these recommendations in Table 9.2 to provide you with some practical tips to use in your mixed methods research practice whenever you evaluate the work of other researchers or plan and implement your own mixed methods study. When you review these recommendations, pay attention to how the authors approach ethical issues and the purposes for using the suggested strategies.

Strategies for managing mixed methods research teams have received more discussion in the mixed methods literature evidently due to increasing numbers of interdisciplinary mixed methods projects. Recommendations to address team dynamics have been developed using different theoretical frameworks, methodological perspectives, and research experiences within and across different disciplines (Creswell et al., 2011; Curry et al., 2012; Hemmings et al., 2013; Johnson et al., 2014). We summarized and discussed these recommendations in Table 9.3 to provide you with some practical tips to use in your mixed methods research practice when you engage in team work with

Table 9.2 Recommendations for Addressing Issues Related to Mixed Methods Research Ethics

Publication	Recommendations for Research Practice	Comments
Creswell, Klassen, Plano Clark, and Smith for the Office of Behavioral and Social Sciences Research (2011)	• Identify and describe issues related to the protection of human subjects. • Understand ethical issues associated with quantitative and qualitative research procedures. • Anticipate ethical issues specifically related to the use of mixed methods. • Be prepared to educate institutional review board (IRB) reviewers about mixed methods research.	These recommendations: • were developed by a team consisting of professionals and academicians writing in the context of health sciences research. • focus on the issues to consider for a National Institutes of Health (NIH) mixed methods research grant application. • are framed from the perspective of methodological diversity for addressing complex health-related issues.
Hesse-Biber (2010b)	• Consider ethical principles guiding your work and life. • Reflect on your ethical obligations to participants. • Consider how your ethical framework and philosophy ensure respect and sensitivity for participants. • Address the ways of communicating to participants the study process, informed consent, and protection of privacy. • Follow the IRB and institutional guidelines, and assess the level of confidentiality for participants. • Consider participants' confidentiality when providing access to data.	These recommendations: • were developed by the author writing in the context of social and behavioral research. • focus on the ethical guideline questions to address for the project. • are framed from the perspective of a reconceptualization of the mixed methods research process through the lens of the qualitative research approach.
Curry and Nunez-Smith (2015)	• Review application instructions to identify requirements unique for qualitative or mixed methods research. • Contact human research protection program staff before submission for guidance on mixed methods protocols. • Communicate clearly and effectively to reviewers defining all terms and using common language and figures. • Seek advice and feedback from a research team or a colleague with expertise in mixed methods.	These recommendations: • were developed by the authors writing in the context of health sciences research. • focus on providing helpful tips for preparing a strong mixed methods research application for human research protection program review. • are framed from the practical perspectives of researchers and reviewers.

Table 9.3 Recommendations for Addressing Issues Related to Mixed Methods Research Team Dynamics

Publication	Recommendations for Research Practice	Comments
Curry, O'Cathain, Plano Clark, Aroni, Fetters, and Berg (2012)	• Deal with differences. • Trust the other. • Create a meaningful group. • Handle conflict and tension. • Enact effective leadership roles within the team.	These recommendations: • were developed by a team consisting of professionals and academicians writing in the context of health sciences and social research. • focus on the challenges to address in mixed methods research teams in the health sciences. • are framed from the representational group theory.
Hemmings, Beckett, Kennerly, and Yap (2013)	• Paradigm level: Generate a shared viewing position through re-education, and construct a theoretical model. • Methods level: Capitalize on members' methodological expertise, and develop effective approaches to combining methods. • Technique level: Develop a new quantitative culture assessment tool to use in combination with complementary qualitative observations and interviews.	These recommendations: • were developed by the authors writing in the context of education and nursing research. • focus on strategies for building an interdisciplinary mixed methods community of research practice at three levels: paradigm, methods, and technique. • are framed from the theories of socialization and organizational culture.

Source	Recommendations	
Creswell, Klassen, Plano Clark, and Smith for the Office of Behavioral and Social Sciences Research (2011)	• Use research questions to determine the expertise required to address them. • Include breadth and depth of methodological expertise. • Transcend distinct methodological and epistemological differences. • Recruit team members with both distinct and interdisciplinary methodological positions and expertise. • Take time to develop the team's capacity. • Demonstrate a history of successful collaboration. • Be experienced and interested in qualitative, quantitative, and mixed methods research. • Create a shared vision and defined roles within the team. • Recognize and honor different team members' perspectives.	These recommendations: • were developed by the authors writing in the context of health sciences research. • focus on strategies for forming and leading successful mixed methods research teams. • are framed from Rosenfield's (1992) taxonomy of three levels of collaboration between social and health scientists.
Johnson, Onwuegbuzie, Tucker, and Icenogle (2014)	• Build a capacity of team members to articulate their philosophy, visions, values, and research goals. • Facilitate group interactions to create conditions for values-sharing dialogue, setting group goals, and developing trust. • Systematically optimize values that support dialectical pluralism conditions and communities of practice.	These recommendations: • were developed by the authors writing in the context of social and behavioral research. • focus on the purposes and strategies for optimizing dialectical pluralism as a foundation for mixed methods teams. • are framed from the dialectical pluralism implementation framework.

other researchers. When you review these recommendations, pay attention to the authors' disciplinary backgrounds and the purposes for applying the suggested strategies.

Despite the challenges that authors may experience with publishing mixed methods research, there is yet limited practical advice about how to deal with these challenges. The emergent discussions address the possible ways of reporting mixed methods studies (Creswell, 2015; Stange, Crabtree, & Miller, 2006), addressing the challenges of the peer review process (Curry & Nunez-Smith, 2015; Dahlberg et al., 2010) and becoming an active co-constructor of quality standards for publishing mixed methods research (Papadimitriou et al., 2013). Along with these discussions, several publications in the JMMR offer practical advice to authors about how to develop publishable mixed methods manuscripts (Creswell & Tashakkori, 2007; Freshwater & Cahill, 2012; Mertens, 2011). We summarized and discussed some of these recommendations for research practice in Table 9.4 to provide you with some practical tips to use in your mixed methods research practice whenever you evaluate published mixed methods research or prepare your own research for publication. When you review these recommendations, pay attention to the authors' disciplinary backgrounds and the specific purposes of the provided guidelines. We also suggest you revisit Table 7.2 in Chapter 7 where we summarized the JMMR guidelines for publishing empirical and methodological mixed methods articles.

ISSUES AND DEBATES ABOUT INTERPERSONAL CONTEXTS AND MIXED METHODS RESEARCH

The emergent literature on the challenges of interpersonal contexts for mixed methods research underscores the importance of acknowledging these issues and generating discussions and potential debates about them for the field to move forward. Here, we introduce some of the issues about interpersonal contexts and mixed methods that form emergent discussions within the field of mixed methods research.

1. How should mixed methods be used to study vulnerable populations? Mixed methods research, reportedly, provides a common language for researchers from different academic disciplines and methodological traditions

Table 9.4 Recommendations for Addressing Issues Related to Editorial and Review Board Guidelines

Publication	Recommendations for Research Practice	Comments
Stange, Crabtree, and Miller (2006)	• Publish quantitative and qualitative papers in separate journals but with clear references and links to other article(s). • Publish concurrent or sequential quantitative and qualitative papers in the same journal. • Publish an integrated single article that describes both methods and findings and draws overarching lessons, with or without appendices that provide study details. • Copublish separate qualitative and quantitative papers accompanied by a third paper that draws overarching lessons from analyses across the two methods. • Develop an online discussion of readers and invited commentators to foster cross-disciplinary communities of knowledge.	These recommendations: • were developed by the authors writing in the context of health sciences research. • focus on providing guidelines for publishing empirical mixed methods studies in health sciences journals. • are framed from the practical perspective of acceptance and recognition of benefits of using mixed methods research in the field of family medicine.

(Continued)

Table 9.4 (Continued)

Publication	Recommendations for Research Practice	Comments
Mertens (2011)	• Include both quantitative and qualitative components and their integration. • Provide a rationale for the use of mixed methods in the study. • Consider your philosophical assumptions and theoretical frameworks. • Include both quantitative and qualitative types of questions. • Be explicit about the sampling strategies that were used for each approach at the planning stage. • Be explicit about what types of data were collected and how they were analyzed. • Provide supportive documentation of the process and outcomes of integrating quantitative and qualitative data. • Be explicit about where in the design the mixing of the methods occurs. • Be cognizant of mixed methods implications at each stage in the research process.	These recommendations: • were developed by the author writing in the context of social and behavioral research. • focus on criteria for publishing high-quality empirical mixed methods studies in the *Journal of Mixed Methods Research* (JMMR). • are framed from the perspective of the editor of the JMMR.

Papadimitriou, Ivankova, and Hurtado (2013)	• Be explicit about the steps in the research process to ensure reviewers can understand and adequately evaluate the study. • Explain how your study uniquely contributes to mixed methods research where consensus does not appear to exist. • Become a reviewer of mixed methods research studies for journals in your field. • Discuss mixed methods research in public venues to promote and educate about it.	These recommendations: • were developed by the authors writing in the context of social and behavioral research. • focus on strategies for co-construction of norms and standards for mixed methods research as determined by scholarly communities. • are framed from the perspective that knowledge is socially constructed and is shaped by a scholarly community.
Creswell (2015)	• Generate three separate papers from a mixed methods study: quantitative, qualitative, and "overall." • Add a methodological paper discussing unique mixed methods procedures. • Target different journals. • Observe the sequence in publishing separate papers. • Provide a "cross-reference" from one paper to another to establish consistency and reduce the length. • Use tables to condense information. • Educate the readers about mixed methods.	These recommendations: • were developed by the author writing in the context of social and health sciences research. • focus on providing guidelines for publishing empirical mixed methods studies to meet journal specifications. • are framed from the perspectives of editor, reviewer, and researcher.

(Continued)

Table 9.4 (Continued)

Publication	Recommendations for Research Practice	Comments
Curry and Nunez-Smith (2015)	• Carefully read and interpret the reviewers' comments. • Outline the major and minor comments received. • Consider if there is an overlap or inconsistency in comments. • Consider if reviewers made erroneous observations or overlooked the content. • In case reviewers lack understanding of mixed methods, clarify and defend the approach in the response letter. • Persuade reviewers that their comments were considered seriously and responded to as appropriate. • Resubmit the revised manuscript before the deadline.	These recommendations: • were developed by the authors writing in the context of health sciences research. • focus on providing guidelines for responding to peer reviews. • are framed from the practical perspectives of researchers and reviewers.

to study vulnerable and marginalized populations (Gomez, 2014; Mertens, 2015). There is consistency among mixed methods researchers about the importance of including participants from at-risk groups, as they provide an insider's view that "richly contributes to the development of more thorough results" (Gomez, 2014, p. 317). Besides, such inclusion helps to balance etic (researchers') and emic (participants') views (Onwuegbuzie & Johnson, 2006) in accurately capturing the experiences and their interpretations that exist within a culture. Mixed methods is also seen as useful because it combines the prolonged community engagement with the advantages of integrating quantitative and qualitative methods (Windsor, 2013). We suggest you refer to multiple examples of mixed methods studies that focused on marginalized populations to identify the best ways to engage these groups in research.

2. **Is using mixed methods research a burden or a benefit to research participants?** There is an emergent discussion about the trade-offs of mixed methods research along with its benefits and advantages for study participants. Mixed methods research may be seen as a burden because it may require more time commitment on the part of research participants, the collection of their identifying information for follow-up purposes, and numerous follow-up contacts that may disrupt their lives (Creswell et al., 2011). Additionally, potential risk associated with collecting both quantitative and qualitative data is doubled in mixed methods studies (Curry & Nunez-Smith, 2015). At the same time, using a mixed methods approach to study an issue may help solicit more information generated from multiple data sources, learn about participants' firsthand experiences, and make them more engaged with the study outcomes (Curry, Nembhard, & Bradley, 2009). Ultimately, using mixed methods research may result in a greater "individual or community impact" (Creswell et al., 2011, p. 24). We suggest you pay attention to the discussion of these issues when you read mixed methods studies to identify the unique burdens and benefits of this approach.

3. **How should researchers adapt reporting a mixed methods study to journal specifications?** Should researchers publish a mixed methods study in its entirety? Dahlberg and colleagues (2010) argued that although a mixed methods study follows the same research steps as a mono-method study, mixed methods researchers have to decide how to organize the presentation of the quantitative and qualitative components to fit the guidelines of the journals in their content areas. Mertens (2011) posited that each researcher should

make this decision "based on the data collection and analysis strategies that were used" (p. 5). However, Cameron (2011) suggested that mixed methods researchers should "develop new ways of thinking about the presentation of research results, especially where the methods used and information gained does not neatly fit a conventional format" (p. 98). There is also consistency in the views that authors should try to adapt their study reporting to the standards of their disciplines and publish separate quantitative and qualitative papers, as well as an "overall" or entire mixed methods study, when needed (Creswell, 2015; Stange et al., 2006). Such an approach may also fit researchers who need to generate multiple publications from a funded mixed methods project. We suggest you study the guidelines for reporting research in your disciplinary journals and also explore how other researchers publish mixed methods studies in your content area to make an informed decision about what approach to take to publish your mixed methods research.

These three questions highlight important issues and debates related to the role of interpersonal contexts in mixed methods research. They also indicate the importance for researchers to identify and recognize the different interpersonal contexts and to find the ways to best address these contexts when engaging in mixed methods research practice.

APPLYING INTERPERSONAL CONTEXTS IN MIXED METHODS RESEARCH PRACTICE

As we outlined in this chapter, interpersonal contexts directly and indirectly influence how researchers approach and use the mixed methods research process in their studies. Because interpersonal contexts play such an important role, understanding their influences is equally imperative for reading and reviewing mixed methods research done by others as well as for proposing and reporting your own mixed methods projects. Box 9.1 includes our advice for applying the concepts of this chapter to your mixed methods research practice.

When you read and review the mixed methods research literature, it is important that you pay particular attention to how interpersonal contexts might have shaped the authors' use and reporting of mixed methods research. We recommend that you first look for explicit statements about how the authors plan to address or addressed the issues related to mixed methods

Box 9.1

Advice for Applying Interpersonal Contexts in Mixed Methods Research Practice

Advice for Reading/Reviewing Mixed Methods Studies and Methodological Discussions

- When reading and reviewing mixed methods research, consider the interpersonal contexts, including mixed methods research ethics, research participant considerations, research team dynamics, and editorial and review board guidelines that might have shaped the authors' use and reporting of mixed methods research.
- Look for statements written by the authors that explicitly identify their approaches for addressing interpersonal contexts and what implications those might have had for the use of mixed methods. If not stated explicitly, look for clues in how the authors considered mixed methods research content and made decisions about a study's research process.
- Assess the extent to which the reported mixed methods study complies with general ethical norms for research and the ethical research standards advanced in the authors' discipline and the mixed methods literature.
- Assess the extent to which the strategies used by the authors to address research participant considerations and team dynamics are consistent with the practical recommendations for dealing with these interpersonal contexts advanced both in the authors' discipline and the mixed methods literature.
- Assess the extent to which the reported mixed methods study is consistent with the conventions for publishing research in the mixed methods field and the authors' discipline.

Advice for Proposing/Reporting/Discussing Mixed Methods Research

- Reflect on interpersonal contexts that you have to consider as you engage in mixed methods research and how they may influence your personal beliefs and methodological considerations.

(Continued)

(Continued)

- Explore the available discussions about interpersonal contexts and practical recommendations for addressing them in your disciplinary and the mixed methods literature, and cite this literature to support your decisions.
- Establish your ethical standpoint from the beginning to control for any misconduct and violation of research ethics advanced in your discipline. Be aware of the ethical issues related to mixed methods research, and consider how to address them.
- Be explicit about how you plan to address or addressed the issues related to engaging participants and other stakeholders in research and to monitoring the team dynamics.
- Explore the editorial and review board guidelines for the journals in your field when you prepare to publish your mixed methods study.

research ethics, research participant considerations, and research team dynamics in their study. If the information is not stated explicitly, reflect on how interpersonal contexts might have influenced the authors' decisions about the study process based on what you have learned from the available discussions in your field and from the mixed methods literature. Be aware that the authors might have used unique approaches not reported in the literature, so be ready to evaluate their relevance in the context of achieving the research purpose—for example, including study participants as co-researchers or providing the local ethical review board with data collection protocols for the study strand that builds on the results from the strand that has not yet been completed. Finally, check the guidelines of the journal that published the mixed methods study, and reflect on how these guidelines, as well as the conventions for publishing research in your discipline, might have influenced the final study report.

It is equally important to consider the role and influences of interpersonal contexts when designing, conducting, and reporting your own mixed methods study. We recommend that you reflect on interpersonal contexts and how they may shape your use of mixed methods at the very onset of your engagement with mixed methods research. We also recommend that you start with exploring the literature in your discipline and the mixed methods field for available discussions and practical recommendations, paying particular attention to how other researchers addressed interpersonal contexts in their research practice. Talk with the representatives of your institution's ethical review board or your colleagues about the ethical issues to envision and deal with when designing and conducting a mixed methods study. If you conduct research in a team, develop a strategy for dealing with the team dynamics to maximize each member's input into the study process. When you report your mixed methods study, be explicit about how you addressed the issues related to interpersonal contexts within the parameters of the journal guidelines.

CONCLUDING COMMENTS

We conclude the chapter by offering some final summary comments organized by the learning objectives stated at the beginning of the chapter.

- **Understand different interpersonal contexts for mixed methods research.** As researchers plan for and implement their mixed methods studies, they enter a complex system of relationships with study participants, co-researchers, and other audiences. These external factors play an important role because they create the power dynamics that influence the mixed methods research process used in a study.
- **Recognize how considerations related to compliance with research ethics, research participants, research team dynamics, and relationships with editorial and review boards shape mixed methods research practice.** These interpersonal considerations form a complex system of relationships that influence researchers' personal contexts in how they apply their beliefs and background knowledge to mixed methods research practice. Likewise, through personal contexts, interpersonal contexts shape researchers' perspectives for each methodological content domain that, in turn, influence and shape the mixed methods research process.
- **Describe practical approaches for addressing interpersonal contexts for mixed methods research.** It is important to understand and find ways to successfully address the influences of interpersonal contexts.

Recommendations for research practice developed from different disciplinary contexts and theoretical backgrounds are available in the mixed methods literature.

APPLICATION QUESTIONS

1. Describe the role of interpersonal contexts in shaping your mixed methods research practice. Discuss why it is important to consider these contexts when engaging in mixed methods research and how they may influence other contexts and methodological domains as outlined in our socio-ecological framework for mixed methods research.

2. Locate a published mixed methods research study from your area of interest and, based on the information included in the article, identify each type of interpersonal contexts (research ethics, research participant considerations, research team dynamics, editorial and review board guidelines) that might have shaped the researchers' use of mixed methods research. Then, discuss what the nature of those influences might have been.

3. Review Tables 9.1 through 9.4 that listed the discussions of interpersonal contexts. Search for a similar discussion of mixed methods research published in your area of interest that addressed examples of interpersonal contexts (mixed methods research ethics, research participant considerations, research team dynamics, and editorial and review board guidelines). What do you conclude about the role of interpersonal contexts in this area based on this discussion? Explain your conclusions.

4. Based on the discussion about interpersonal contexts you located for Question 3, describe the recommendations for research practice that are advanced in the literature in your field. What other potential strategies to deal with or account for those issues can you suggest based on the information highlighted in the chapter?

5. Pick one of the ongoing issues and debates about interpersonal contexts for mixed methods highlighted in this chapter. State why you selected that issue, and discuss your reactions to this issue in terms of its importance for mixed methods research practice. Do you think this issue warrants further discussion or debate?

KEY RESOURCES

To learn more about interpersonal contexts for mixed methods research, we suggest you start with the following resources:

  *1. Marti, T. S., & Mertens D. M. (Eds.) (2014). Special issue: Marginalized populations. *Journal of Mixed Methods Research, 8*(3), **207–321.**

  - This volume of the JMMR is devoted to the issues of engaging the underserved and vulnerable populations in research, using a transformative mixed methods approach. The collection of articles illustrates four main methodological strategies aimed at the inclusion of these populations and soliciting their voices and insights.

  2. Hesse-Biber, S. N. (2010). The centrality of ethics in the mixed methods research process. In *Mixed methods research: Merging theory with practice* (pp. 55–59). New York, NY: Guilford Press.

  - In this chapter, Hesse-Biber discussed ethical dilemmas specific to mixed methods research as they relate to different stages of a mixed methods study. She also offered ethical questions to guide researchers in conducting their mixed methods projects.

  *3. Creswell, J. W., Klassen, A. C., Plano Clark, V. L., & Smith, K. C. for the Office of Behavioral and Social Sciences Research. (2011). The protection of human subjects. In *Best practices for mixed methods research in the health sciences* (pp. 23–24). Bethesda, MD: National Institutes of Health.

  - In this section of the report, Creswell and colleagues provided a list of ethical issues for researchers to anticipate and address when developing a mixed methods research proposal in the health sciences.

  *4. Curry, L. A., O'Cathain, A., Plano Clark, V. L., Aroni, R., Fetters, M., & Berg, D. (2012). The role of group dynamics in mixed methods health sciences research teams. *Journal of Mixed Methods Research, 6*(1), 5–20.

  - In this article, Curry and colleagues explored the dynamics of mixed methods research teams; discussed the challenges related to organizational, professional, and individual differences of team members;

and offered some principles to guide mixed methods research teams in the health sciences.

* The key resource is available at the following website: http://study.sagepub.com/planoclark.

⁂ TEN ⁂

HOW DO SOCIAL CONTEXTS SHAPE MIXED METHODS?

CONSIDERING INSTITUTIONAL, DISCIPLINARY, AND SOCIETAL INFLUENCES ON MIXED METHODS RESEARCH

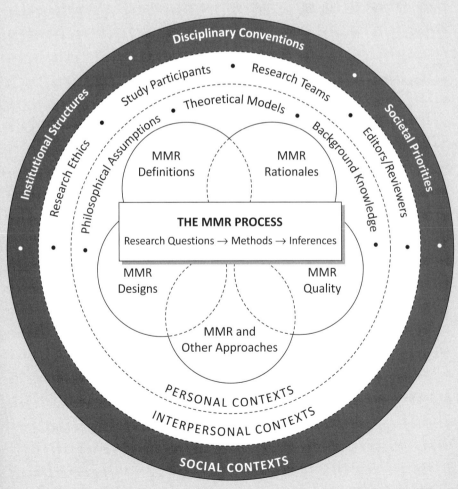

247

*T*he final category of contexts for mixed methods research practice that we consider is social contexts. When you engage in mixed methods research practices as a scholar, researcher, reviewer, or instructor, you do so within a certain environment shaped by your many social contexts. These environments include your academic institutions; disciplinary research communities; and local, regional, and national settings. Social contexts provide significant influences on the use of mixed methods research; therefore, they merit important consideration within the field. In addition to shaping the mixed methods research content considerations and research process, social contexts play a notable role by influencing interpersonal and personal contexts for mixed methods research. In this chapter, we discuss several perspectives and debates about social contexts to help you understand their importance for mixed methods research. We also include examples and recommendations for addressing personal contexts in mixed methods research practice.

LEARNING OBJECTIVES

This chapter aims to provide you with an understanding of social contexts that shape mixed methods content considerations and the research process so you are able to do the following:

- Recognize different social contexts for mixed methods research.
- Understand how institutional, disciplinary, and societal contexts shape mixed methods research practice.
- Describe how the status of mixed methods research is considered within different social contexts.

CHAPTER 10 KEY CONCEPTS

The following key concepts will help you navigate through the main considerations related to social contexts for mixed methods research as they are introduced in this chapter:

- **Social contexts:** The institutional structures, disciplinary conventions, and societal priorities that shape mixed methods research practice.

- **Institutional contexts:** Structures within professional settings, including how mixed methods is taught and promoted within academic programs, that shape mixed methods research practice.
- **Disciplinary contexts:** Conventions held by communities of research practice, including preferences for certain research questions and approaches, that shape mixed methods research practice.
- **Societal contexts:** Priorities within society-defined groupings, including national values and funding policies, that shape mixed methods research practice.
- **Status of mixed methods research:** The extent to which mixed methods research is used and perceived to be accepted as an approach to research within a specific community of researchers.

THE ROLE OF SOCIAL CONTEXTS IN THE FIELD OF MIXED METHODS RESEARCH

Throughout this book, we have considered mixed methods research practice and how the field of mixed methods research has advanced different perspectives for the mixed methods research process, content considerations, and personal and interpersonal contexts that shape this practice. We have now reached the outermost level of our socio-ecological framework for mixed methods research, which we identify as social contexts. **Social contexts** are the institutional structures, disciplinary conventions, and societal priorities that shape mixed methods research practice. For example, as a student in an academic program, you experience the influence of institutional structures that determine whether and what kind of coursework on mixed methods research is offered. As a member of a certain discipline, you learn about disciplinary conventions for the acceptability of the mixed methods approach to research. As a member of a specific society, you are also subject to the influence of priorities and policies set by entities at the local and national levels, such as whether funding agencies support mixed methods research. Collectively, these social contexts interact with each other to provide the environment in which you engage in mixed methods research, and ultimately this environment influences how you approach mixed methods research practice.

Keep in mind that social contexts play an influential role in *all* research. For example, research is often impacted by policies established by the larger society. If you conduct a study in the field of education, your research will likely be influenced by policies that mandate curricular priorities and testing procedures. Although influences such as these are found in all forms of research, our intention here is to focus on the influential social contexts for mixed methods research. By placing social contexts in the outermost level of our model as depicted in Figure 10.1, we highlight the importance of social contexts specifically for mixed methods research practice. As Figure 10.1 suggests, social contexts influence researchers' interpersonal and personal contexts for mixing methods. For example, national policies regarding research ethics shape researchers' interactions with human subject review boards

Figure 10.1 The Role of Social Contexts in the Practice of Mixed Methods Research

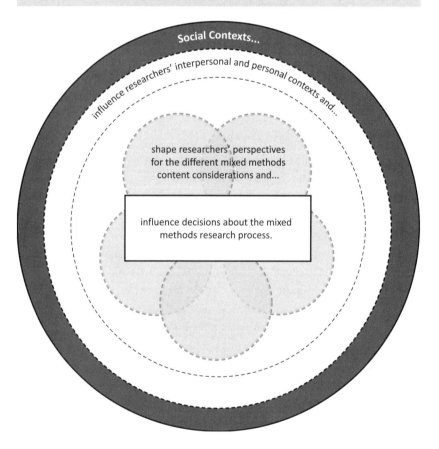

regarding their use of mixed methods research. Disciplinary norms regarding acceptable research methods influence the background knowledge that researchers bring to the use of mixed methods. Social contexts also shape the mixed methods research content considerations, such as when disciplinary conventions suggest which mixed methods definition to follow or what quality standards are considered appropriate. In addition, we find that social contexts can directly influence researchers' decisions about the mixed methods research process. For example, funding parameters might dictate which research questions are worth seeking answers to or academic program expectations might require that one method (quantitative or qualitative) be prioritized over the other. Because of the pervasive nature of social contexts, their implications are an essential element to fully understand mixed methods research practice.

MAJOR PERSPECTIVES ABOUT SOCIAL CONTEXTS FOR MIXED METHODS RESEARCH

The development of the field of mixed methods research has been profoundly shaped by, and therefore concerned with, the social contexts in which scholars consider and apply mixed methods research. Many of the earliest writings in the field examined the application and implications of mixing methods within specific research communities and social contexts (e.g., Greene, Caracelli, & Graham, 1989), often with an aim to advance understanding and support of this research approach within the community. Although all research is shaped by social contexts, their influence is particularly salient for new, emergent research methodologies such as mixed methods because new methodologies need to be understood within, adapted to, and accepted by existing social contexts (Hesse-Biber & Leavy, 2008; Morgan, 2007; Plowright, 2011). In some situations, social contexts serve to constrain the use of mixed methods, such as by discounting it as a legitimate form of research or limiting the types of mixed methods approaches that are viewed as acceptable within a discipline. In other situations, social contexts support and encourage the use of mixed methods, such as by promoting it as a preferred research approach. In either case, when scholars review, write about, propose, discuss, or report the use of mixed methods research, they craft their work based on socially constructed conventions and to satisfy the expectations of specific audience groups. To help you understand the major perspectives about these complex influences, we highlight three broad (and interrelated) types of social contexts discussed in the mixed methods literature: institutional, disciplinary, and societal contexts.

Institutional Contexts

As you consider the social contexts that influence your approach to mixed methods research, you likely first think of influences from your graduate program such as the methodological expertise of the members of the faculty, the research methods courses available and/or required, and the types of faculty recruited to teach in your program. These are examples of institutional contexts. **Institutional contexts** are the structures within professional settings, including how mixed methods is taught and promoted within academic programs, that shape mixed methods research practice. Relevant parameters related to academic programs include whether the program favors either a quantitative or a qualitative research approach; whether or not mixed methods is taught; and if it is taught, whether it is introduced throughout the program or as a specialized advanced topic. Although not limited to academic programs, it is the structure of academic programs and the teaching of mixed methods specifically that has received the most attention in the literature thus far. This is likely because of their influence on researchers' use of mixed methods and because the incorporation of formal coursework can serve as an indicator for the larger acceptance of mixed methods research (Plano Clark, 2005).

The teaching of formal mixed methods courses has been identified as particularly challenging due to the emergent nature of the field (Creswell, Tashakkori, Jensen, & Shapley, 2003; Greene, 2010; Tashakkori & Teddlie, 2003b; Teddlie & Tashakkori, 2010). This emergent nature means that the mixed methods research content considerations are still unsettled and debated (as we emphasized in Chapters 3 through 7) and that currently few instructors received formal coursework in mixed methods during their own graduate training so they have few models for structuring their own courses. There is, however, a growing literature on instructors' experiences to guide thinking about teaching mixed methods research within academic programs (e.g., Baran, 2010; Christ, 2009, 2010; Ivankova, 2010; Ivankova & Plano Clark, 2014, 2015; Leech & Onwuegbuzie, 2010; Onwuegbuzie, Frels, Collins, & Leech, 2013; Poth, 2014). Examining these writings identifies several facets that vary across mixed methods courses, including the instructional format (e.g., face-to-face or distance learning), the required prerequisite courses (e.g., quantitative and qualitative research), the course pedagogical features (e.g., objectives, textbooks, additional readings, schedules of topics, and assignments), the course emphasis (e.g., supplementing quantitative or qualitative methods, designing a mixed methods study, or introducing mixed methods perspectives and debates), and the number and sequence of mixed methods courses required (e.g., one semester, two semesters, or throughout the program). These facets serve to distinguish the different experiences that students have when completing mixed methods coursework and the different decisions that instructors make when teaching mixed methods courses.

Disciplinary Contexts

Along with considering the level of institutionalization of mixed methods research within your academic program, another key social context that you likely readily identify is your research discipline. Your research discipline is the substantive content area in which you work and it represents the community of scholars who serve as the primary audience for your scholarship. Disciplines can be viewed as very broad (e.g., education, health sciences, or psychology) or more narrow and specialized (e.g., adolescent development, public health, or career development). **Disciplinary contexts** are the conventions held by communities of research practice, including preferences for certain research questions and approaches, that shape mixed methods research practice. As such, your disciplinary contexts shape the training you receive, the research problems that you address, the terminology you use, the conferences you attend, and the journals in which you disseminate your scholarship.

With the great differences that exist among our substantive disciplines, it is no wonder that there are great variations in the disciplinary contexts that exist for mixed methods and the ways in which mixed methods is discussed and applied (Denscombe, 2008; Tashakkori & Creswell, 2008). In some disciplines, the use of mixed methods is ubiquitous and unremarkable compared to other research approaches, but in other disciplines, it is exotic, unusual, or even discouraged (Alise & Teddlie, 2010; Ivankova & Kawamura, 2010; Plano Clark, 2005). Disciplinary contexts for mixed methods have been examined in many ways in the literature, such as in terms of the types of research questions and theories that are used (e.g., Rudd & Johnson, 2010; Stentz, Plano Clark, & Matkin, 2012), the dominant method priority and paradigms (e.g., Alise & Teddlie, 2010; Ross & Onwuegbuzie, 2012), the historical developments and trends (e.g., Small, 2011), and the prevailing attitudes about mixed methods (e.g., Roberts & Povee, 2014). A discipline's conventions for mixed methods can often be described in terms of the acceptability, prevalence, and typical use of mixed methods by researchers who are trained and publishing within the discipline.

Societal Contexts

The third type of social context that we highlight is societal contexts. **Societal contexts** are priorities within society-defined groupings, including national values and funding policies, that shape mixed methods research practice. Consider the society-defined groupings that might influence your mixed methods research practice. These often include organizations and agencies at the local, regional, or national levels that support the production of research. These groups, including governmental agencies and nongovernmental organizations, are involved with research through policy initiatives that shape priorities for research and/or by directly funding research endeavors. As with the institutional and disciplinary contexts, societal contexts represent different levels of support for and acceptance of the use of mixed methods research.

Within the mixed methods literature, societal contexts have often been considered in terms of national settings for the use of mixed methods, particularly as they relate to national funding for research. Scholars have examined and described the level of support for mixed methods within national contexts such as the United States (Plano Clark, 2010), Canada (Islam & Oremus, 2014), and the United Kingdom (O'Cathain, Murphy, & Nicholl, 2007). While Western countries such as these are described as becoming generally supportive of mixed methods research, scholars are also beginning to examine the emergent presence of mixed methods within other national contexts such as France (Dupin, Debout, & Rothan-Tondeur, 2014), East China (Zhou & Creswell, 2012), and Nigeria (Dumbili, 2014). These writings note varying levels of support for mixed methods and identify important contexts for ensuring this support, such as how academic training is provided within the national context. Even within a specific context, scholars find that societal contexts are complex and nuanced. For example, within the United States, Saint Arnault and Fetters (2011) described how their planned use of mixed methods received enthusiastic support from the federal funding source, but Christ (2014) described how current national funding priorities in the United States limit researchers' use of mixed methods. Likewise, when mixed methods studies are successfully funded by national entities, that funding can still constrain researchers' use of mixed methods. For instance, Canadian researchers Miall and March (2005) noted that the choice of their mixed methods design was impacted by their national funding agency. They explained, "We had intended to draw an interview sample from the larger telephone survey. In reviewing our research proposal, the funding agency mandated a qualitative study followed by a survey" (p. 407).

CONSIDERING THE STATUS OF MIXED METHODS RESEARCH WITHIN SOCIAL CONTEXTS

Because of their powerful influences, social contexts have been of great interest to researchers using mixed methods research throughout the development of the field. Much of this work has focused on the **status of mixed methods research,** which is the extent to which mixed methods research is used and perceived as an accepted and supported form of research within specific research communities. The status of mixed methods is important because it indicates whether specific research communities are knowledgeable about mixed methods, are using mixed methods to address important research problems, and are willing to support and fund mixed methods applications. As you engage in mixed methods research practice as a researcher, scholar, and reviewer, it can be very useful to consider the literature about the status of mixed methods research within your research community. There are three broad types of publications that you may encounter about the status of mixed methods. We refer to these publications as advocacy writings, systematic methodological reviews, and disciplinary-based discussions of mixed methods research, and we introduce their primary features in the paragraphs that follow.

Advocacy writings are publications in which authors provide an introduction to mixed methods research to a particular research community and argue for the merit and value of its use specifically for members of that community. Advocacy writings typically define mixed methods research, review its historical development, summarize different possible approaches and designs, and provide a few notable exemplars of the use of mixed methods from within the community. In general, authors develop advocacy writings with the explicit intent of enhancing the status of mixed methods within their research communities by increasing awareness of mixed methods and helping to legitimize this approach through a prestigious publication. Therefore, advocacy writings are particularly influential when they are published in important journals within the field. For example, Johnson and Onwuegbuzie (2004) published their advocacy piece within the *Educational Researcher,* a premier journal in the field of education. Its influence within the field of education has been remarkable, as best indicated by the high number of citations the article has received in the 10 years since its publication (more than 5,000 citations according to Google Scholar). Advocacy writings have appeared in a wide variety of fields to date, and the number continues to increase as more scholars choose to advocate for the legitimacy and acceptance of mixed methods research within specific communities. We provide a few select examples of advocacy writings in Table 10.1, although many more such publications exist. Writings such as these are particularly useful for you to cite when proposing or reporting a mixed methods study in a field where the use of mixed methods is currently relatively uncommon.

Another way that scholars consider the status of mixed methods research is to conduct *systematic methodological reviews.* In disciplinary-based systematic methodological reviews, scholars systematically examine researchers' use of mixed methods within one (or more) social context to identify trends and patterns about that use. When you read a systematic methodological review, you notice that the authors report having used methodical procedures for identifying a sample of published mixed methods studies and reviewing specific dimensions and features reported within those publications. Examples of mixed methods dimensions that are reviewed within such publications include the rationale for mixing methods; the timing, integration, and priority of the methods in the mixed methods research process; and the type of mixed methods design used. In addition, some systematic methodological reviews specifically consider additional dimensions such as the prevalence rate and citation impact of the use of mixed methods as compared to the use of quantitative and qualitative research approaches. There is a long history of scholars conducting disciplinary-based methodological reviews in the field of mixed methods research to learn about researchers' use of mixed methods. Early reviews included fields such as evaluation (Greene et al., 1989), nursing (Swanson, 1992), higher education (Creswell, Goodchild, & Turner, 1996), primary medical care (Creswell, Fetters, & Ivankova, 2004), and counseling

Table 10.1 A Few Select Examples of Advocacy Writings for Mixed Methods Research

Publication	Discipline	Mixed Methods Topics Discussed	Comments
Grafton, Lillis, and Mahama (2011)	Accounting research	• Defining and describing mixed methods research • Rationales for mixing methods • The risks of mixing methods • Examples of mixed methods studies from the field	• An advocacy writing for a field that already makes extensive use of both quantitative and qualitative research
Curry, Nembhard, and Bradley (2009)	Cardiovascular disease research	• Defining qualitative and mixed methods research, including when and how to use them • Examples of qualitative and mixed methods research from the field • Quality considerations for qualitative and mixed methods research • Future directions for using qualitative and mixed methods research to study cardiovascular diseases	• An advocacy writing in a field that makes extensive use of quantitative research
Johnson and Onwuegbuzie (2004)	Education research	• Historical development of mixed methods research • Pragmatism • Comparison of quantitative, qualitative, and mixed methods research • Mixed methods design typologies and elements • Mixed methods research process • Expected future developments for mixed methods in the field of education	• An advocacy writing in a field concerned about philosophical assumptions for research

(Continued)

Table 10.1 (Continued)

Publication	Discipline	Mixed Methods Topics Discussed	Comments
Bradt, Burns, and Creswell (2013)	Music therapy research	• Need for mixed methods to answer complex questions relevant to the field • Core characteristics of mixed methods • Examples of the use of the basic mixed methods designs • Quality criteria for mixed methods research • Recommendations for applying mixed methods in the field	• An advocacy writing in a field that traditionally values quantitative research
Kroll and Neri (2005)	Rehabilitation nursing research	• Need for mixed methods within the field • Introduction to the basic mixed methods designs • How to plan and conduct mixed methods research • Value of mixed methods for rehabilitation nursing research	• An advocacy writing that emphasizes the utility of mixed methods to address the content of interest to the field
Rudd and Johnson (2010)	Sport management research	• Need for mixed methods to address causal research questions of interest to the field • Historical development of mixed methods • Mixed methods designs and procedures • Examples of the use of mixed methods to understand causation	• An advocacy writing tailored to a specific type of research question of primary interest to the field

psychology (Hanson, Creswell, Plano Clark, Petska, & Creswell, 2005). Table 10.2 summarizes several recent (2007–2014) examples of systematic methodological reviews that scholars have conducted to learn about the status of mixed methods within a variety of disciplines. Reviews such as these provide a current picture of the status of mixed methods within a particular context as well as information about how mixed methods is used in that context. Furthermore, some scholars are beginning to conduct cross-disciplinary reviews of the use of mixed methods (Alise & Teddlie, 2010; Ivankova & Kawamura, 2010), which facilitate comparisons between different disciplines. By reading systematic methodological reviews, you can learn about the current conventions for using mixed methods within specific fields, identify good models from within the field, and cite the review to support your use of mixed methods within your disciplinary context.

The third category of publications that speaks to the status of mixed methods research within a specific community is disciplinary-based discussions of mixed methods research. *Disciplinary-based discussions of mixed methods research* are how-to writings where authors offer specific guidelines and recommendations for mixed methods research tailored to a particular community of research practice. That is, instead of writing about mixed methods in general, these writings focus specifically on how mixed methods can and should be adapted and used within a specific discipline. To date, there are several examples of disciplinary-based discussions of mixed methods found in the health sciences. For example, Curry and Nunez-Smith (2015) authored a book that provides a full introduction to mixed methods research written in the context of the health sciences, using language, priorities, and examples drawn from the field. Other examples of disciplinary-based discussions of mixed methods research from the health sciences include a document offering "best practices for mixed methods research" commissioned by the National Institutes of Health (NIH; Creswell, Klassen, Plano Clark, & Smith for the Office of Behavioral and Social Sciences Research, 2011) and an edited volume on consideration and applications of mixed methods in the nursing and health sciences (Andrew & Halcomb, 2009). These types of publications are indicative of mixed methods research having obtained a generally high level of acceptance within the health sciences. Other examples of disciplinary-based discussions of the practice of mixed methods research include the application of mixed methods in teaching English as a second language (Brown, 2014), in criminal justice and criminology (Lanier & Briggs, 2013), and in policy research and evaluation (Burch & Heinrich, 2015). We expect that many more

Table 10.2 Examples of Recent Disciplinary-Based Systematic Methodological Reviews of the Use of Mixed Methods Research

Publication	Discipline	Mixed Methods Dimensions Considered	Other Dimensions Considered	Comments

Jang, Wagner, and Park (2014)	Applied linguistics	• Rationale
		• Timing
		• Mixing
		• Synergistic effects
			• Participants
			• Language content
			• Testing validity issues
			• Collaboration
				• Review scope:
				  ○ 7 databases, 2007–2013
				  ○ $N = 32$ mixed methods articles
				• Results indicated that the use of mixed methods is increasing, occurs for a variety of rationales, and is often related to issues of validity within the studies.

Molina-Azorín (2011)	Business management	• Priority
		• Timing
		• Rationales
			• Prevalence rates
			• Citation impact
				• Review scope:
				  ○ 4 journals, 1997–2007
				  ○ $N = 152$ mixed methods articles
				• Results indicated that mixed methods articles had greater impact than other research articles.

Ross and Onwuegbuzie (2012)	Education	• Priority	• Prevalence rates
			• Content topics and research contexts
				• Review scope:
				  ○ 2 journals, 1999–2008
				  ○ $N = 110$ mixed methods articles
				• Results indicated a high prevalence rate for mixed methods within education (24%) and within math education in particular (33%).

Study	Discipline	Characteristics		Review scope

Plano Clark, Huddleston-Casas, Churchill, Green, and Garrett (2008)	Family sciences	• Language
		• Design types
		• Timing
		• Priority
		• Integration
		• Logistical issues
			• Author national affiliations
			• Content topics
			• Prevalence rates
				• Review scope:
				  ○ 4 journals, 1996–2005
				  ○ N = 19 mixed methods articles
				• Results indicated the use of a variety of designs and several issues related to procedures and context that influenced the use of mixed methods.

O'Cathain, Murphy, and Nicholl (2007)	Health services	• Rationales
		• Qualitative strand methods
		• Quantitative strand methods
		• Priority
		• Timing
			• Prevalence rates
			• Funding programs
				• Review scope:
				  ○ HSR-funded projects in the United Kingdom, 1994–2004
				  ○ N = 75 mixed methods studies
				• The authors also interviewed 20 researchers
				• Results indicated a strong prevalence (18%) for mixed methods projects and emphasized the influence funding priorities have in choosing to use mixed methods.

Stentz, Plano Clark, and Matkin (2012)	Leadership	• Level of interaction
		• Priority
		• Timing
		• Mixing
			• Use of theory
			• Type of participants
			• Author national affiliations
				• Review scope:
				  ○ 1 journal, 1990–2012
				  ○ N = 15 mixed methods studies
				• Results indicated limited but growing use of mixed methods by international researchers in the field.

Harrison and Reilly (2011)	Marketing	• Priority
		• Timing
		• Design type and variant
			• Research purposes	• Review scope:
				  ○ 9 journals, 2003–2009
				  ○ N = 43 mixed methods studies
				• Results indicated limited but growing use of mixed methods and the need for more awareness of the field of mixed methods.

(Continued)

Table 10.2 (Continued)

Publication	Discipline	Mixed Methods Dimensions Considered	Other Dimensions Considered	Comments

Hart, Smith, Swars, and Smith (2009)	Mathematics education	• Qualitative strand methods
		• Quantitative strand methods
		• Priority
		• Integration
			• Prevalence rates	• Review scope:
				  o 6 journals, 1995–2005
				  o $N = 207$ articles that combined qualitative methods and statistical results
				• Results noted a high prevalence for mixed methods approaches (29%) but the need for increased sophistication in the use and reporting of mixed methods.

Cameron (2010)	Vocational education and training	• Integration
		• Rationale
		• Design type
		• Priority
			• Prevalence rates of type of paper
			• Data collection methods
			• Data analysis techniques
				• Review scope:
				  o 2 conferences, 2007–2008, and 1 journal, 2003–2008
				  o $N = 23$ papers that used mixed methods
				• Results noted an overall low prevalence (15%) and quality concerns for mixed methods approaches, with mixed methods more prevalent in conference papers than journal articles.

such publications will be forthcoming in a variety of disciplines as its status continues to grow and expand.

ISSUES AND DEBATES ABOUT SOCIAL CONTEXTS AND MIXED METHODS RESEARCH

Considering the many different disciplines using mixed methods research and its global presence, it is not surprising that we have considered so many different perspectives for and about mixed methods research throughout this book. Although there is general agreement about the importance of social contexts for mixed methods research, there are still ongoing issues and debates related to the issues raised in this chapter. Here, we identify three issues that are discussed and debated within the field.

1. How should mixed methods research be taught? There is general agreement of the value of formal training in mixed methods research, and more and more academic programs are offering coursework and experiences in mixed methods research. However, differing opinions can be found about how best to structure this formal training as part of academic programs. For example, some academic programs emphasize providing a strong foundation in both quantitative and qualitative methods (e.g., Baran, 2010), others provide explicit instruction on mixed methods research (e.g., Ivankova, 2010), and still others argue for teaching all data collection and analysis methods within a mixed research framework (e.g., Onwuegbuzie, Leech, Murtonen, & Tähtinen, 2010). Although there is likely no one best way to teach mixed methods research, as a student or instructor in an academic program, you should be aware of different approaches and strive to continually evaluate and improve the quality and availability of mixed methods training opportunities provided within your program.

2. What is the status and acceptance of mixed methods research? As this chapter has highlighted, an ongoing issue for the use of mixed methods research is its status within specific research communities. Across the literature (and among colleagues), you can find a wide range of opinions and descriptions of the status of mixed methods research. These range from dire warnings (e.g., "mixed methods is not accepted and cannot get funded or published") to extreme claims (e.g., "only proposals for mixed methods studies can get funding"), and every perception between. The key is to recognize that the status of mixed methods research varies and continues to evolve and expand across institutions, disciplines, and nations. You should therefore carefully examine the status of mixed methods research within your own specific social context through the literature and your own experiences so that you can thoughtfully argue for and report about your use of mixed methods research in ways that address the expectations found within your context.

3. Do mixed methods scholars represent their own community of research practice? Through the early history of the field of mixed methods research, the primary concern about social contexts was how they impact mixed methods research practices. As the field has matured, however, a new question is emerging for debate regarding whether mixed methods has become its own distinct research community (Tashakkori, 2009). Although many writings, including this book, highlight the many debates and lack of consensus that exist in the field, there are also many indications of the existence of a productive and thriving community of scholars, which supports the existence of the Mixed Methods International Research Association and several interest groups within other organizations, several journals, and a regular major mixed methods international conference. As you consider this debate in relation to your own social contexts for using mixed methods, consider how connected you are to scholars who share the conventions, priorities, and beliefs that have been discussed throughout this book.

These questions highlight three ongoing conversations within the field about social contexts for mixed methods research. They also point to the important role that our institutional, disciplinary, and societal contexts place on our research in general and use of mixed methods research in particular. The differing opinions that exist acknowledge that social contexts can be both facilitators and barriers to the use of mixed methods research, and successful scholars need to be able to recognize, adapt to, and possibly challenge and change social contexts to conduct the research that they feel is most needed to address important research problems.

APPLYING SOCIAL CONTEXTS IN MIXED METHODS RESEARCH PRACTICE

Whether you engage in advocating for, teaching, planning, conducting, disseminating, or evaluating mixed methods research, your research practice is shaped by your larger environments in the form of social contexts. For better or worse, these contexts provide the settings in which mixed methods research occurs. Although the literature agrees on the importance and relevance of these contexts, there are great variations within the contexts depending on one's institution, discipline, society, and the interactions among these entities. Therefore, it is important for you to consider social contexts and recognize the ways in which they may influence your and others' use of mixed methods research. In Box 10.1, we offer some general advice for considering the concepts of this chapter as they relate to your mixed methods research practice.

One of the best ways to learn about social contexts is to attend to them as you read about and review examples of mixed methods research. When reading

---

Box 10.1

Advice for Applying Social Contexts in Mixed Methods Research Practice

Advice for Reading/Reviewing Mixed Methods Studies and Methodological Discussions

- Recognize that all scholars who engage in mixed methods research practices are situated within their own social contexts (i.e., institutional, disciplinary, and societal contexts).
- When reading about and reviewing mixed methods research, identify the authors' social contexts including their academic institutions, disciplines, funding support, and national affiliations.
- Consider the extent to which the social contexts provided a supportive and/or constraining environment for the authors' use of mixed methods.
- Pay attention to the ways in which the authors' mixed methods research process, content considerations, and personal and interpersonal contexts were shaped by social contexts.
- Assess the extent to which the authors explained how social contexts influenced their mixed methods research practice.
- Assess the extent to which the authors' use of mixed methods was consistent with the structures, conventions, and priorities associated with their social contexts.

(Continued)

(Continued)

Advice for Proposing/Reporting/Discussing Mixed Methods Research

- Reflect on your institutional, disciplinary, and societal contexts as you first consider the use of mixed methods and consider how these social contexts may support or constrain your mixed methods research practice.
- Assess the status of mixed methods research within your social contexts as discussed in writings about mixed methods research, and cite this literature to support your use of mixed methods.
- If needed, take steps to improve the status of mixed methods within your research community, such as by developing advocacy writings or a systematic methodological review.
- When appropriate, shape your use of mixed methods to align with the conventions and priorities associated with your social contexts. When this alignment is not appropriate for your mixed methods research practice, fully justify and explain why your use of mixed methods differs from these conventions and priorities.
- When social contexts directly shape your mixed methods research process and content considerations, explain how and why these influences occurred.

and reviewing mixed methods literature, note the institutional, disciplinary, and societal contexts identified by the authors and consider in what ways they influenced the authors' use of mixed methods and to what extent the authors discussed and explained these influences. Recognize that the way the authors thought about, used, and reported mixed methods likely depends at least to some extent on the prevalence of, conventions for, and opinions toward mixed methods within those social contexts.

It is also important to consider the social contexts in which you work when you conceptualize, design, and report your own mixed methods study. By assessing and reflecting on the status of mixed methods research, you are better able to argue for and position your use of mixed methods in ways that will be understandable and acceptable for the social groups that are the primary audiences for your work. On the one hand, if the status of mixed methods is at the ground level in your setting, then you can expect to need to define this approach in basic terms and explain why it is appropriate for your context. Citing literature such as advocacy writings from within the field can help to bolster your arguments. On the other hand, if mixed methods research has a well-established status in your setting, then you can expect your audience to be knowledgeable and prepared to apply high-quality standards to reviewing your approach. In this case, you should situate your use of mixed methods within ongoing discussions and examples of its use found within the field. The key is to both understand your social contexts and give them critical consideration when proposing, reporting, and discussing mixed methods research.

CONCLUDING COMMENTS

We conclude the chapter by offering some final summary comments organized by the learning objectives stated at the beginning of the chapter.

- **Recognize different social contexts for mixed methods research.** Social contexts represent the environment in which scholars conduct their mixed methods research practice. It is useful to think of these contexts in terms of structures found in academic institutions and programs, conventions and norms established by disciplines, and priorities and policies set by agencies and governments.

- **Understand how institutional, disciplinary, and societal contexts shape mixed methods research practice.** Social contexts influence mixed methods research practice by providing environments with differing levels of acceptance of and support for mixed methods research in terms of the available formal training, the relative preference for the use of mixed methods for addressing disciplinary research problems, and the availability of funding for mixed methods research. These environments influence how researchers learn about, use, assess, and discuss mixed methods research.

- **Describe how the status of mixed methods research is considered within different social contexts.** The status of mixed methods research within a particular social context is often described in terms of the prevalence of and perceived level of acceptance for the use of mixed methods research by the corresponding community. The status within specific social contexts is often examined and promoted through advocacy writings, systematic methodological reviews, and disciplinary-based discussions published in the literature.

APPLICATION QUESTIONS

1. Locate a published mixed methods research study from your area of interest and, based on the information included in the article, identify the social contexts that might have shaped the researchers' use of mixed methods research. Discuss what the nature of those influences might have been.

2. Locate a discussion of mixed methods research published in your area of interest that is an example of an advocacy writing, systematic methodological review, or disciplinary-based discussion. What do you conclude about the status of mixed methods research in this area based on this discussion? Explain your conclusions.

3. Describe your perceptions of the status of mixed methods research within your institutional contexts, such as whether certain methods are favored, expertise in mixed methods is present, and formal coursework in mixed methods is available. Discuss how this environment might influence your use of mixed methods research.

4. Describe your perceptions of the status of mixed methods research within your disciplinary contexts, such as the extent to which members of your discipline are knowledgeable about mixed methods and the prevalence of the use of mixed methods research within the field. Discuss how this environment might influence your use of mixed methods research.

5. Describe your perceptions of the status of mixed methods research within your societal contexts, such as the extent to which mixed methods research aligns with current funding priorities. Discuss how this environment might influence your use of mixed methods research.

6. Pick one of the ongoing issues and debates about social contexts for mixed methods: when and how mixed methods research should be taught, whether the use of mixed methods research is accepted or not,

or if there is a community of mixed methods researchers. State why you selected that issue, and discuss your reactions to this issue in terms of the environment for the use of mixed methods research.

KEY RESOURCES

To learn more about social contexts for mixed methods research, we suggest you start with the following resources:

1. **Onwuegbuzie, A. J., Frels, R. K., Collins, K. M. T., & Leech, N. L. (2013). Conclusion: A four-phase model for teaching and learning mixed research. [Editorial].** *International Journal of Multiple Research Approaches,* **7**(1), 133–156.

   - In this article, Onwuegbuzie and colleagues reviewed many of the decisions and challenges associated with teaching mixed methods research at the graduate level. They also described their own approach to teaching mixed methods, which is organized by a model of the research process that includes four phases: conceptual/theoretical, technical, applied, and emergent scholar.

*2. **Alise, M. A., & Teddlie, C. (2010). A continuation of the paradigm wars? Prevalence rates of methodological approaches across the social/behavioral sciences.** *Journal of Mixed Methods Research,* **4**(2), 103–126.

   - In this article, Alise and Teddlie presented a systematic methodological review of the use of mixed methods across four prominent disciplines (education, nursing, psychology, and sociology) to highlight disciplinary differences in the status and use of mixed methods research.

*3. **Plano Clark, V. L. (2010). The adoption and practice of mixed methods: U.S. trends in federally funded health-related research.** *Qualitative Inquiry,* **16**(6), 428–440.

   - In this article, Plano Clark summarized the importance of social contexts for mixed methods research and then presented a systematic methodological review of mixed methods proposals that received federal funding in the health sciences within the United States.

*4. **Tashakkori, A. (2009). Are we there yet? The state of the mixed methods community [Editorial].** *Journal of Mixed Methods Research, 3*(4), 287–291.

  - In this editorial, Tashakkori provided his reflections on the existence of a distinct community of mixed methods scholars that can provide a social context for conducting mixed methods research.

  * The key resource is available at the following website: http://study.sagepub.com/planoclark.

PART IV

CONCLUDING THOUGHTS

You have now completed your examination of the different components of our socio-ecological framework for the field of mixed methods research organized by the mixed methods research process, content, and contexts. For each component, we introduced you to the different perspectives, debates, and issues found within the field of mixed methods research. From these discussions, you have now developed a solid understanding of mixed methods research, which will help you navigate the mixed methods field. This understanding should play an important role when you advocate for the use of mixed methods within your research environments; plan, implement, and disseminate mixed methods studies to address your research questions; evaluate the use of mixed methods by others; and learn and share knowledge about mixed methods research with others. Therefore, in this final part of the book, we offer our concluding thoughts about how you can continue to apply the framework for the field of mixed methods research within your current or future mixed methods research practice. The chapter in Part IV is as follows:

Chapter 11: Where Is Mixed Methods Research Headed? Applying the Field in Your Mixed Methods Research Practice

WHERE IS MIXED METHODS RESEARCH HEADED?

APPLYING THE FIELD IN YOUR MIXED METHODS RESEARCH PRACTICE

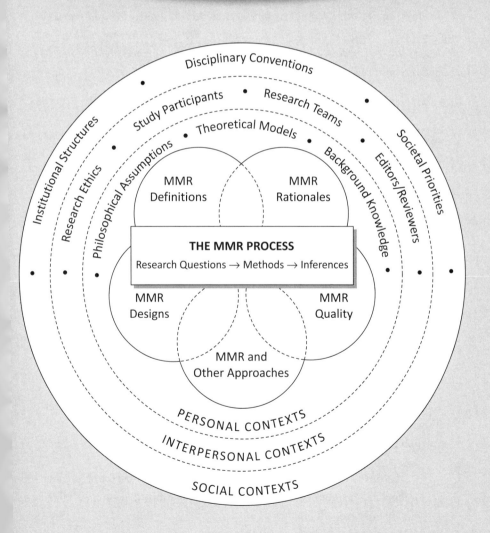

*B*y completing the previous chapters of this book, you have examined the field of mixed methods research in terms of each of the levels and components within our socio-ecological framework. Our goal for this final chapter, therefore, is to step back and help you consider the entire framework more holistically, including how you might continue to apply the framework to guide your understanding and applications of the field of mixed methods research in your research practice. We start this chapter by examining the complexity of mixed methods research practice as demonstrated by the interactions within and among the components of the mixed methods research process, content considerations, and contexts. From there, we offer our recommendations for applying the framework as you continue with your learning about and use of mixed methods research. We conclude this chapter by describing our reflections about future directions for the field of mixed methods research.

LEARNING OBJECTIVES

This chapter aims to provide you with an understanding of how you can further apply the field of mixed methods research to your research practice so you are able to do the following:

- Recognize the complexity inherent within mixed methods research.
- Apply the socio-ecological framework for mixed methods research to your learning about and use of mixed methods.
- Contemplate future directions for the field of mixed methods research.

CHAPTER 11 KEY CONCEPTS

The following key concepts will help you navigate through the main considerations related to understanding and applying the field of mixed methods research as they are introduced in this chapter:

- **Messiness of mixed methods research:** A concept used to recognize the inherent complex, dynamic, and undetermined nature of mixed methods research practice.

- **Process-oriented approach to mixed methods research:** An approach to discussing mixed methods research framed by the general steps in the process of research in which researchers consider the foundations for their study, state a research purpose and questions, choose a design, implement methods, draw inferences, ensure quality, and disseminate study results.
- **Methodologically oriented approach to mixed methods research:** An approach to discussing mixed methods research framed by philosophical, theoretical, and/or logistical considerations.
- **Future developments for mixed methods research:** The advancements that will continue to occur in our understanding of the mixed methods research process, content considerations, and contexts in terms of the philosophical, theoretical, methodological, and technical aspects of examining and using mixed methods research.

UTILITY OF OUR SOCIO-ECOLOGICAL FRAMEWORK TO GUIDE YOUR MIXED METHODS RESEARCH PRACTICE

As first discussed in Chapter 1, we conceptualized the field of mixed methods research in terms of the socio-ecological framework in response to our own understanding of the field and to facilitate our goals for teaching about mixed methods research in formal courses and informal research consultations. As highlighted throughout this book, we consider this framework to be a useful guide for conceptualizing the primary concepts in the field of mixed methods research and recognizing the diverse perspectives, including debates and issues within those perspectives, that convey the richness and nuances of the field. By examining these points across the ten previous chapters, you now have a good introduction and solid foundation in understanding the field of mixed methods research and its implications for mixed methods research practice.

Although our focus in this book has been on using this framework to introduce the field of mixed methods research, we have found that its utility goes beyond organizing the topics in this book. We regularly use this framework to conceptualize how the mixed methods research literature can inform and guide our thinking about our mixed methods research practice as scholars, researchers, reviewers, and instructors. In this chapter, therefore, we discuss four different ways that you might continue to apply the framework to guide

your understanding and application of the field of mixed methods research in
your research practice:

- To understand the complexity of mixed methods research studies
- To design and implement mixed methods research studies
- To develop further expertise in mixed methods research
- To identify future directions for mixed methods research

APPLYING THE FRAMEWORK: UNDERSTANDING THE MESSINESS OF MIXED METHODS RESEARCH

All models and frameworks are attempts to understand and explain some complex aspects or phenomena of the world. We developed our framework for
describing the field of mixed methods research with this purpose in mind. First
of all, we wanted to understand the field of mixed methods research that has
become quite messy and difficult to navigate. Second, we wanted to find a way
to communicate this messiness to our students and colleagues to enhance their
process of applying mixed methods in their research practice. We believe that
approaching complex phenomena, such as the field of mixed methods research,
from the socio-ecological perspective that underscores the interconnectedness
and interrelatedness of ideas, is effective to assist in understanding and presenting
the current status of mixed methods research. Therefore, our goal for using the
socio-ecological framework in this book has been to provide a model of the field
of mixed methods research that facilitates understanding and applying the key
elements and diverse perspectives that make up the field. We believe that the
framework serves this purpose well, but we also recognize that the field is very
complex, dynamic, and fluid and therefore cannot be fully understood as neatly
falling within the nine components included in the three levels of the framework.
Furthermore, as we attempted to show in the book, there is a constant interaction
between the levels and domains in the framework that contributes to the complexity and messiness of the field. Therefore, it is important to consider the
messiness inherent within mixed methods research and how the socio-ecological
framework can help you identify and understand sources of messiness.

Messiness of mixed methods research is a concept found in the literature that recognizes the inherent complex, dynamic, and undetermined nature

of mixed methods research practice (Freshwater, 2007; Seltzer-Kelly, Westwood, & Peña-Guzman, 2012). Mixed methods research practice is inherently complex due to the inclusion of multiple perspectives and approaches. It is also inherently dynamic as the combination of scholars' multiple perspectives and approaches leads to new insights and tensions in the expressed ideas and in the outcomes of research. Moreover, mixed methods research practice is inherently undetermined because those insights and tensions cannot be fully anticipated or predicted. Many sources of messiness in mixed methods research arise from the interactions that occur among the contexts, content considerations, and research process found within mixed methods research practice. Therefore, our socio-ecological model can also help you identify and understand this messiness.

The mixed methods research literature has devoted increasing attention to not only describing but even calling for increased acknowledgment of and reflection about the messiness of mixed methods research (e.g., Freshwater, 2007; Freshwater & Fisher, 2014). As an example of answering this call, Seltzer-Kelly and colleagues (2012) described the "multiplicity and messiness" (p. 258) of their experiences in conducting their mixed methods educational research study in which they attempted to "quantitize" qualitative results as part of their research process. Their article highlights how this mixed methods research process interacted with their mixed methods content considerations and contexts in unexpected and profoundly important ways. Content considerations highlighted in their discussion included their rationale of complementarity for mixing the methods, their planned design and its emergent features, and their attempt to apply quality criteria based on quantitative validity standards to the quantitizing process. The contextual influences experienced within their study included each researcher's individual philosophical beliefs, theoretical orientations, and prior experiences related to the research topic; the interactions that occurred among the team members around their different roles (e.g., student, faculty member) and assumptions about research; and the disciplinary and funding pressures encouraging the use of mixed methods research. Seltzer-Kelly and colleagues described how they collectively grappled with the interactions among these many elements as they worked to apply good research practices discussed in the mixed methods literature in their mixed methods study.

As another example of the messiness of mixed methods research, Campbell, Patterson, and Bybee (2011) told the "tale" of their experiences and challenges in conducting a sequential mixed methods study about sexual assault survivors. Notable interactions occurred among the considerations related to their research process, content domains, and contexts that contributed to the messiness of their use of mixed methods. Examples of their study's messiness included the interactions among funding pressures, disciplinary expectations for research, their research questions, their choice of a sequential Quan → Qual design, the sequential timing of the research process, the individual researchers' different philosophical assumptions and prior training, the use of different theoretical perspectives, and the interactions with different types of participants (e.g., police, prosecutors, and survivors). In their article, Campbell and colleagues (2011) highlighted the complexity of mixed methods research and the tensions inherent in a research approach that purposefully brings together multiple perspectives, approaches, and contexts. By recognizing that many of these tensions arise in the interactions both within and among the levels of the socio-ecological framework, you can better understand this "messiness" and thoughtfully consider its role within mixed methods research practice.

APPLYING THE FRAMEWORK: IMPLEMENTING YOUR MIXED METHODS RESEARCH STUDIES

Unquestionably, it is beneficial for you to be able to understand and describe the messiness inherent within mixed methods research as a contemporary scholar, but if you are reading this book, you are likely particularly interested in applying its ideas as you navigate the implementation of mixed methods research to study research questions of interest to you. The implementation of a mixed methods research study requires you to make many decisions about your approach to mixed methods research and the procedures you will use to address your research purpose. In order to successfully navigate these complex decisions, it is essential for you to connect the knowledge developed in the field of mixed methods research to the decisions you make as you plan, conduct, and report your research. Therefore, in this section, we explicitly consider how you can apply the framework advanced in this book to the steps of study planning and implementation.

Fortunately, there is much guidance available in the literature for the steps required to plan and implement a mixed methods research study, and the key concepts introduced in this book will serve as a strong foundation from which you can carefully consider the many decisions required. Many of the available writings in the field of mixed methods research are organized using a process-oriented approach (e.g., Creswell & Plano Clark, 2011; Greene, 2007; Teddlie & Tashakkori, 2009). When scholars follow a **process-oriented approach to mixed methods research,** they frame their discussions of mixed methods research using the general steps in the process of research. Although a variety of terminology is used, these steps typically include researchers considering the foundations for their study, stating a research purpose and questions, choosing a design, implementing methods, drawing inferences, ensuring quality, and disseminating study results. When applied to mixed methods research, these steps direct the decisions involved in planning and conducting a mixed methods study. To illustrate a process-oriented approach to mixed methods, we briefly discuss two examples of the steps required when implementing a mixed methods research study as outlined in the literature.

The first example of the steps required to implement a mixed methods research study comes from Collins and O'Cathain (2009). These authors offered 10 key points for planning a mixed methods study for novice researchers who are new to mixed methods research. We have listed these 10 steps in the first two columns of Table 11.1. Collins and O'Cathain noted that these steps related specifically to the phases of formulating the research (Steps 1–5), planning the research (Steps 6–7), and implementing the research (Steps 8–10). Taken together, these 10 points provide a useful set of guidelines to help novice researchers with conducting a mixed methods study. In addition, each of the steps requires decisions about the mixed methods research process that are informed by mixed methods research content considerations and are shaped by contexts. Therefore, in the last column of Table 11.1, we note which components of the socio-ecological framework are emphasized within each of the 10 points. For example, the first steps of defining mixed methods research and being aware of your mental model for mixing methods directly relate to the components of mixed methods research definitions and mixed methods research personal and social contexts. You should note that each component of the field of mixed methods research is directly related to one or more of the steps in the study process.

Table 11.1	Applying the Socio-Ecological Framework to Collins and O'Cathain's (2009) Recommended Points to Consider for Novice Researchers Implementing a Mixed Methods Research Study

Step	Collins and O'Cathain's (2009) Points Organized by the Research Process	Application of the Socio-Ecological Framework Components
1	Define mixed methods research.	*MMR Content:* • MMR definitions
2	Be cognizant of your mental model (i.e., assumptions, values, and experiences) for mixing.	*MMR Contexts:* • Personal contexts • Social contexts
3	Utilize typologies of mixed methods research designs to provide overall guidelines.	*MMR Content:* • MMR designs • MMR intersecting with other approaches
4	Select the reason, rationale, and purpose for mixing.	*MMR Content:* • MMR rationales
5	Determine the research question.	*MMR Process:* • Research questions
6	Develop the mixed methods research design.	*MMR Process:* • Methods *MMR Content:* • MMR designs • MMR intersecting with other approaches
7	Determine the sampling design.	*MMR Process:* • Methods *MMR Contexts:* • Interpersonal contexts
8	Collect data from participants.	*MMR Process:* • Methods *MMR Contexts:* • Interpersonal contexts
9	Conduct data analysis.	*MMR Process:* • Methods
10	Legitimate inferences and formulate generalizations.	*MMR Process:* • Inferences *MMR Content:* • MMR quality

NOTE: MMR = mixed methods research.

As a second example of applying the framework to the implementation of a mixed methods study, Table 11.2 lists seven steps for developing a mixed methods study that Creswell, Klassen, Plano Clark, and Smith for the Office of Behavioral and Social Sciences Research (2011) suggested for health sciences researchers who are new to mixed methods research. These steps describe the research process from a study's conceptualization through report writing. Once again, we have linked each of these steps to the corresponding components of our socio-ecological framework, which are listed in the last column of Table 11.2. Although there are some differences in the order and content of the steps provided in the two tables, you should again note that all of the components of the framework relate to these important steps. Keep in mind that mixed methods research is complex (as discussed earlier in this chapter) and process-oriented approaches are useful simplifications of the inherent messiness. Therefore, the elements listed in Tables 11.1 and 11.2 emphasize only the most salient steps and components and not the interactions among them. When implementing a mixed methods study, it is helpful to be guided by a clear set of process steps but to also reflect about the messiness of that process as it is experienced.

If you plan to implement a mixed methods research study in your areas of interest, we strongly recommend that you choose at least one resource organized by a process-oriented approach to help you work through the steps of study planning and implementation. There are many quality books available that discuss the steps of mixed methods research from the perspective of the research process. Table 11.3 (see page 284) lists eight prominent books using a process-oriented approach to mixed methods that we recommend as quality resources for applying the field of mixed methods research to the steps required to implement mixed methods in your research study. For each resource, we provide a list of the chapter topics to convey an overview of its research-process approach as well as our commentary about the books' emphasis and social contexts. Based on the reactions we have heard from students and colleagues over the years, we also note the audiences for which the book typically has a general appeal. These resources are all practical in nature and present discussions of mixed methods from a single, consistent perspective (representing one or two authors). We encourage you to review the list and select at least one or two books that seem to best align with your perspectives and contexts for using mixed methods research to inform your application of mixed methods in a research study.

Table 11.2   Applying the Socio-Ecological Framework to Creswell et al.'s (2011) Major Steps to Consider for Researchers Developing a Funding Proposal to Implement a Mixed Methods Research Study

Step	Creswell et al.'s (2011) Steps Organized by the Research Process	Application of the Socio-Ecological Framework Components
1	Consider your philosophy, theory, resources, research problem, and reasons for using mixed methods.	*MMR Contexts:* • Personal contexts • Interpersonal contexts • Social contexts *MMR Content:* • MMR definitions • MMR rationales
2	State aims and research questions that call for qualitative, quantitative, and mixed methods research and incorporate your reasons for using mixed methods.	*MMR Process:* • Research questions *MMR Content:* • MMR rationales
3	Determine the timing, priority, and integration for your qualitative and quantitative methods of data collection and analysis.	*MMR Process:* • Methods
4	Select a mixed methods design.	*MMR Content:* • MMR designs • MMR intersecting with other approaches
5	Collect and analyze the data.	*MMR Process:* • Methods *MMR Contexts:* • Interpersonal contexts
6	Interpret how the combined results address the research problem and research questions.	*MMR Process:* • Inferences *MMR Content:* • MMR quality
7	Write the final report.	*MMR Contexts:* • Interpersonal contexts • Social contexts

NOTE: MMR = mixed methods research.

APPLYING THE FRAMEWORK: DEVELOPING
YOUR EXPERTISE IN MIXED METHODS RESEARCH

When engaging in mixed methods research practice, it is important to balance the voice of a single perspective (such as found in the books listed in Table 11.3) with the many different perspectives that coexist in the field of mixed methods research. Therefore, although books that take a process-oriented approach to mixed methods research are very useful for working through the steps of implementing a mixed methods study, they cannot adequately represent the many different perspectives and continuing advancements occurring in the field. In order for your mixed methods research practice to be as rigorous and current as possible, it is important for you to connect with the mixed methods literature to continue learning about the methodological issues salient for mixed methods research.

A good way to further develop your expertise for mixed methods research is to read literature that takes a more methodologically oriented approach to mixed methods in addition to the literature that presents a process-oriented approach. We think of a **methodologically oriented approach to mixed methods research** as an approach where authors discuss mixed methods research framed by philosophical, theoretical, and/or logistical considerations. Methodologically oriented approaches to mixed methods research may focus on the full scope of mixed methods research (as we have attempted to do in this book) or may focus on a specific and narrow aspect of mixed methods research (such as the options and implications of sampling decisions in mixed methods). Because of the diversity of topics and perspectives found in methodologically oriented writings about mixed methods research, it may be useful to keep our socio-ecological framework in mind as you read such resources. By attending to how the readings relate to the framework, you will be well positioned to understand where a particular topic fits within the larger field, consider how it relates to the mixed methods research process, and recall what other perspectives exist about the topic.

In Table 11.4, we provide a list of several key sources of methodologically oriented approaches to mixed methods research. The items listed in the table are all edited sources that represent the perspectives of many different scholars on many different mixed methods research topics, as highlighted in the provided overviews and our comments. Note that several of the listed sources

Table 11.3 Select Examples of Recent Books That Examine Mixed Methods Research From a Process-Oriented Approach

Book	Chapters	Comments
Creswell and Plano Clark (2011)	1. The Nature of MMR 2. The Foundations of MMR 3. Choosing a MM Design 4. Examples of MM Designs 5. Introducing a MM Study 6. Collecting Data in MMR 7. Analyzing and Interpreting Data in MMR 8. Writing and Evaluating MMR 9. Summary and Recommendations	• *Emphasis:* Practical method considerations for using MM throughout the process of research for specific MM designs • *Social contexts:* Authors from the United States and the field of education • *General appeal:* Researchers wanting a step-by-step discussion of using MM
Curry and Nunez-Smith (2015)	1. Definition and Overview of MM Designs 2. Applications and Illustrations of MM Health Sciences Research 3. Determining the Appropriateness and Feasibility of Using MM 4. Writing a Scientifically Sound and Compelling Grant Proposal for a MM Study 5. Examples of Funded Grant Applications Using MM 6. Assessing Quality in MM Studies 7. Sampling and Data Collection in MM Studies 8. Data Analysis and Integration in MM Studies 9. Managing MM Teams 10. Implementation Issues in MMR 11. Publishing MM Studies in the Health Sciences	• *Emphasis:* Practical considerations for using MM in the context of the health sciences • *Social contexts:* Authors from the United States and in the field of health sciences • *General appeal:* Pragmatic health science researchers wanting practical guidance on design and logistical issues for using MM

| Greene (2007) | 1. Mental Models and MM Inquiry
2. Adopting a MM Way of Thinking
3. The Historical Roots of the Contemporary MM Conversation
4. Contested Spaces: Paradigms and Practice in MM Social Inquiry
5. Stances on Mixing Paradigms and Mental Models While Mixing Methods
6. Mixing Methods on Purpose
7. Designing MM Studies
8. MM Data Analysis
9. Judging the Quality of MM Social Inquiry
10. Writing up and Reporting MM Social Inquiry
11. The Potential and Promise of MM Social Inquiry | • *Emphasis:* Philosophical and methodological considerations for using MM
• *Social contexts:* Author from the United States and the field of evaluation
• *General appeal:* Philosophically oriented researchers wanting thoughtful guidance for why and how to use MM |
| Hesse-Biber (2010b) | 1. Introduction to MMR
2. Formulating Questions, Conducting a Literature Review, Sampling Design, and the Centrality of Ethics in MMR
3. A Qualitative Approach to MM Design, Analysis, Interpretation, Write Up, and Validity
4. Interpretive Approaches to MMR
5. Feminist Approaches to MMR
6. Postmodernist Approaches to MMR
7. Putting It Together: Qualitative Approaches to MMR Praxis
8. Conclusion: The Prospects and Challenges of MM Praxis | • *Emphasis:* Interpretive and critical perspectives for using MM
• *Social contexts:* Author from the United States and in the field of sociology and women's studies
• *General appeal:* Qualitatively and transformative-oriented researchers wanting discussions of how to apply MM |

(Continued)

Table 11.3 (Continued)

Book	Chapters	Comments
Ivankova (2015)	1. Introducing MMR 2. Introducing Action Research 3. Applying MM in Action Research 4. Conceptualizing a MM Action Research Study 5. Designing a MM Action Research Study 6. Planning Integration of Quantitative and Qualitative Methods in a MM Action Research Study 7. Sampling and Collecting Data in a MM Action Research Study 8. Analyzing Data in a MM Action Research Study 9. Assessing Quality of a MM Action Research Study 10. Planning and Implementing Action Using MM Action Research Study Inferences	• *Emphasis:* Considerations for intersecting MMR with an action research methodological approach • *Social contexts:* Author from Ukraine and the United States and in the field of education and health sciences • *General appeal:* Action-oriented researchers wanting a rigorous MM approach within an action research study
Morgan (2014)	1. An Introduction and Overview 2. Pragmatism as a Paradigm for MMR 3. Research Design and Research Methods 4. Motivations for Using MMR 5. The Sequential Priorities Model 6. Preliminary Qualitative Inputs to Core Quantitative Research Projects 7. Preliminary Quantitative Inputs to Core Qualitative Research Projects	• *Emphasis:* Practical considerations for sequential MM approaches • *Social contexts:* Author from the United States and in the field of sociology • *General appeal:* Pragmatically oriented researchers and researchers wanting to use sequential MM designs

	8. Follow-up Qualitative Extensions to Core Quantitative Research Projects 9. Follow-Up Quantitative Extensions to Core Qualitative Research Projects 10. Multipart Sequential Designs 11. Finding the Expertise to Combine Multiple Methods 12. Conclusions: Further Thoughts About Research Design	
Morse and Niehaus (2009)	1. MM Design: Who Needs It? 2. The Nuts and Bolts of MM Design 3. Theoretical Drive 4. Pacing the Components 5. The Point of Interface 6. Sampling for MM Designs 7. Planning a MM Project 8. Qualitatively-Driven MM Designs 9. Quantitatively-Driven MM Designs 10. Complex Mixed and Multiple Method Designs	• *Emphasis:* Considerations for theoretically driven MM designs • *Social contexts:* Authors from Canada and in the field of nursing and education • *General appeal:* Researchers using inductive or deductive approaches to combine two or more quantitative and/or qualitative methods

(Continued)

287

Table 11.3 (Continued)

Book	Chapters	Comments
Teddlie and Tashakkori (2009)	1. MM as the Third Research Community 2. The Fundamentals of MMR 3. Methodological Thought Before the 20th Century 4. Methodological Thought Since the 20th Century 5. Paradigm Issues in MMR 6. Generating Questions in MMR 7. MMR Designs 8. Sampling Strategies for MMR 9. Considerations Before Collecting Your Data 10. Data Collection Strategies for MMR 11. The Analysis of MM Data 12. The Inference Process in MMR	• *Emphasis:* Pragmatic foundations for MM to develop strong inferences • *Social contexts:* Authors from the United States and Iran and in the field of social psychology and education • *General appeal:* Pragmatic and quantitatively oriented researchers

NOTE: MM = mixed methods; MMR = mixed methods research.

Table 11.4 Select Examples of Key Edited Sources That Offer Methodologically Oriented Discussions About Mixed Methods Research

Edited Source	Description	Comments

Bergman (2008)	• 11 chapters organized in two major sections:
	  o The Theory of MM Design
	  o Applications in MM Design
		• Examination of MMR in the context of the social sciences by 20 scholars from the United States and Europe

Hesse-Biber and Johnson (2015)	• 40 chapters organized in five major sections:
	  o Linking Theory and Method
	  o Conducting MMR
	  o Contextualizing MMR
	  o Incorporating New Technologies in MMR
	  o Commentaries About MMR
		• Comprehensive examination of MMR in the context of the social and health sciences by 68 scholars from North America, Europe, and Australasia

Journal of Mixed Methods Research (JMMR) (Sage; 2015 Editors: Freshwater & Fetters)	• Peer-reviewed journal published on a quarterly basis starting in January 2007 (http://mmr.sagepub.com)	• New contributions to the field of MMR across diverse disciplines and national contexts
International Journal of Multiple Research Approaches (Taylor & Francis; 2015 Editor: Grbich)	• Peer-reviewed journal published two times per year starting in January 2007 (http://www.tandfonline.com/loi/rmra)	• New contributions to the field of MMR across diverse disciplines and national contexts

(Continued)

Table 11.4 (Continued)

Edited Source	Description	Comments
Mixed Methods Research Series (Sage, 2015; Editors: Plano Clark & Ivankova)	• Series of books published on an intermittent basis (about one to three per year) starting in 2015 (www.sagepub.com/mmrs)	• In-depth practical guidance for specific MMR topics across diverse disciplines and national contexts

Plano Clark and Creswell (2008)	• 23 chapters organized in two major sections:
	  ○ Methodological Selections
	  ○ Exemplar Research Studies
		• Selected collection of reprinted mixed methods discussions and examples by 52 scholars from different disciplines, nations, and time periods (1979–2007)

Tashakkori and Teddlie (2003a)	• 26 chapters organized in four major sections:
	  ○ The Research Enterprise in the Social and Behavioral Sciences: Then and Now
	  ○ Methodological and Analytical Issues for MMR
	  ○ Applications and Examples of MMR Across Disciplines
	  ○ Conclusions and Future Directions
		• Comprehensive examination of MMR in the context of the social and health sciences by 52 scholars from North America, Europe, and Australia

Tashakkori and Teddlie (2010b)	• 31 chapters organized in three major sections:
	  ○ Conceptual Issues: Philosophical, Theoretical, Sociopolitical
	  ○ Issues Regarding Methods and Methodology
	  ○ Contemporary Applications of MMR
		• Comprehensive examination of MMR in the context of the social and health sciences by 52 scholars primarily from North America, Europe, and Australia

NOTE: MM = mixed methods; MMR = mixed methods research.

are ongoing journal or book publications, which means that they will continue to offer new perspectives and topics as the field continues to evolve and develop. Indicative of the growing interest in mixed methods across specific disciplines, there is also an increasing number of edited books that provide methodologically oriented discussions of mixed methods research within a particular content area. Examples include edited volumes about the use of mixed methods research in the topic areas of child development (Weisner, 2005); nursing and health sciences (Andrew & Halcomb, 2009); stress and coping in education (Collins, Onwuegbuzie, & Jiao, 2010); and physical education, sports, and dance (Camerino, Castañer, & Anguera, 2012). These are particularly useful volumes to learn about mixed methods research when they directly relate to your own areas of interest. We strongly recommend that you seek out and read different sources about mixed methods research that present a variety of perspectives and contexts to expand your expertise in mixed methods research.

APPLYING THE FRAMEWORK: FUTURE DEVELOPMENTS IN MIXED METHODS RESEARCH

A final way that we suggest you apply the framework for the field of mixed methods research is to help you identify future developments for the field that are needed and/or anticipated. By **future developments for mixed methods research,** we mean the advancements that will continue to occur in our understanding of the mixed methods research process, content considerations, and contexts. Therefore, future developments will include advancements in terms of the philosophical, theoretical, methodological, and technical aspects of examining and using mixed methods research. There have been numerous calls for new developments in the field to address many of the ongoing debates and issues that exist and that we have highlighted throughout this book (e.g., Creswell, 2010; Greene, 2008; Hesse-Biber & Johnson, 2013; Mertens, 2013; Tashakkori & Teddlie, 2010a). Future developments arise as scholars work to address knowledge gaps that exist in the field of mixed methods research. Therefore, many mixed methods research studies have the potential to contribute to our understanding of mixed methods research if the researchers are able to identify ways in which their research practices are novel and could contribute to the mixed methods literature. Considering your mixed methods research practice in relation to the larger field may help you identify ways in which your own scholarship could advance understanding of mixed methods research (in addition to your content area of interest).

As we write this final chapter of this book, we are eager to see what advancements in the field of mixed methods research will occur in the years ahead. As researchers, we continually examine our own use of mixed methods and consider whether there is potential for future developments from this work. As methodologists, we dedicate our methodological scholarship to identifying gaps in knowledge and advancing understanding of those gaps. As instructors, we encourage our students to look for innovative ways of applying mixed methods to their unique research situations. Finally, as editors, we seek new works that will contribute to the field. Throughout these various activities, we also find it useful to apply our framework for the field to consider and organize potential future developments. Although no one can predict what advancements will emerge in the future, here we offer a few reflections about our expectations for future directions for mixed methods research within each level of our framework.

Future Developments About the Mixed Methods Research Process

There is great potential for future developments in the field of mixed methods research that will advance our understanding of research purpose and questions, methods, and inferences that make up the mixed methods research process. For example, the field has only begun to fully examine the range of research questions that can best be answered using mixed methods research and the types of inferences that can be drawn from integrated results as well as how those questions and inferences interact with certain mixed methods research content and context considerations. In addition, we anticipate extensive future developments in terms of the conceptual and technical aspects of the methods used in the mixed methods research process. Examples of such developments will likely include innovative sampling procedures; new strategies for effectively integrating quantitative and qualitative components of a study; procedures for incorporating additional dimensions within the integration such as biological measures, time, or levels of a system; secondary data analysis of existing quantitative and qualitative databases; and application of multimedia tools to facilitate integration such as creative use of existing tools or development of new software tools.

Future Developments About Mixed Methods Research Content

Our understanding of the major content considerations for mixed methods research will also continue to be enhanced through future developments. For example, quality standards for mixed methods will continue to be refined in general but also further adapted to the considerations involved in certain mixed methods designs or from particular foundational assumptions. We anticipate many future developments related to mixed methods research designs—particularly in terms of the implications for when researchers intersect basic mixed methods designs with other methodological approaches and frameworks. Likewise, future work may carefully examine the connections among mixed methods definitions, rationales, quality, basic designs, and their intersections with other approaches to further untangle these considerations and suggest ways in which they need to be congruent with each other.

Future Developments About Mixed Methods Research Contexts

Much work is still needed in understanding, problematizing, and strategizing about contexts for mixed methods research. This work includes further consideration about how to adapt mixed methods research practice to certain contexts. Examples of such developments might include guidance for how graduate programs can best prepare scholars to become mixed methods researchers and how researchers should tailor their use of mixed methods to meet the expectations of audiences such as dissertation committees, funding agencies, and journal reviewers. Further work is definitely needed that carefully examines the ethical aspects of conducting mixed methods research and ethical implications for the kinds of research questions that are asked, the role of participants in mixed methods research studies, and the way that mixed methods research is reported. In addition, future developments need to also consider ways in which researchers can effectively challenge, change, and resist contexts that serve to limit and constrain the use of mixed methods research.

Although there is a need for future developments within each of the levels of our framework for the mixed methods field, some of the most interesting developments will be those that cut across multiple levels and directly address the inherent messiness of mixed methods research. For example, we anticipate further examination and examples of how a certain set of personal philosophical assumptions interacts with specific mixed methods content considerations, such as defining mixed methods and quality considerations as well as the implications of these interactions for a study's mixed methods research process. We look forward to reading and learning about all of these developments—along with many that we do not yet anticipate—in the years ahead!

CONCLUDING COMMENTS

We conclude the chapter by offering some final summary comments organized by the learning objectives stated at the beginning of the chapter.

- **Recognize the complexity inherent within mixed methods research.** Although frameworks such as the one advanced in this book provide a useful organizational structure for examining mixed methods research, it is important to keep in mind that all such frameworks are simplifications of the actual dynamic and interactive systems that they represent. Mixed methods research practice is particularly complex, dynamic, and unsettled—that is, messy—because it purposefully brings together multiple perspectives and approaches. Therefore, its complexity demands considerations for the many components involved in that research practice as well as the interactions among those components.

- **Apply the socio-ecological framework for mixed methods research to your learning about and use of mixed methods.** The framework advanced in this book has great utility for understanding the field of mixed methods research and can help you to apply the knowledge about the field to your mixed methods research practice. Use the framework and your understanding of its components as a foundation for examining the steps involved in planning and implementing a mixed methods research study and for continuing to develop your expertise with mixed methods research.

- **Contemplate future directions for the field of mixed methods research.** Although the field of mixed methods research has become increasingly sophisticated and organized since the late 1980s, there is still the need for much more work to be done! Future developments will focus on gaps within the field of mixed methods research that exist both within the elements of the field as well as the interactions among the elements. As you engage in mixed methods research practice, consider in what ways your work could also contribute to advancing the field.

APPLICATION QUESTIONS

1. Locate a published mixed methods research study from your area of interest. Based on the information included in the article, describe any "messiness" that occurred within the authors' mixed methods research practice and discuss how such messiness supports the complex and dynamic nature of the mixed methods research field.

2. Choose one of the books listed in Table 11.3. Review the titles of the chapters and, based on the information, apply the socio-ecological framework for mixed methods research and note which components of the field of mixed methods research you expect to find emphasized within each of the chapters (as was done in Tables 11.1 and 11.2).

3. Review the major books that discuss the process of conducting mixed methods research as listed in Table 11.3. Select one or two of these books that you would be most inclined to examine to further inform your use of mixed methods research, and explain why you are drawn to those particular books.

4. Consider how you will continue to learn about mixed methods research in order to advance your understanding of and skills for the use of mixed methods research. Write a plan delineating three to five steps that you will take to keep abreast of the field and its developments.

5. Based on the information we presented in this book, what future directions do you feel are most needed in the field of mixed methods research? Explain why you feel these potential developments are needed and why these topics are of interest to you.

KEY RESOURCES

To learn more about how you might further apply the field of mixed methods research to your research practice, we suggest you start with the following resources:

*1. Campbell, R., Patterson, D., & Bybee, D. (2011). Using mixed methods to evaluate a community intervention for sexual assault survivors: A methodological tale. *Violence Against Women, 17*(3), 376–388.

- In this article, Campbell and colleagues recounted the "tale" of the messiness of their use of mixed methods research to study survivors of sexual assault. Their tale highlighted how the authors navigated the dynamic interactions that occurred among their research process; mixed methods design; and personal, interpersonal, and social contexts.

*2. **Seltzer-Kelly, D., Westwood, S. J., & Peña-Guzman, D. M. (2012). A methodological self-study of quantitizing: Negotiating meaning and revealing multiplicity.** *Journal of Mixed Methods Research,* **6(4), 258–274.**

- In this article, Seltzer-Kelly and colleagues described the messiness they experienced in their use of mixed methods research in a diversity curriculum efficacy study. Their reflective self-study reported how the authors navigated the dynamic interactions that occurred among their mixed methods research process, content considerations, and contexts as they implemented an intercoder reliability procedure as part of their data transformation technique.

3. **Collins, K. M. T., & O'Cathain, A. (2009). Ten points about mixed methods research to be considered by the novice researcher.** *International Journal of Multiple Research Approaches,* **3, 2–7.**

- In this article, Collins and O'Cathain presented 10 key ideas that need to be considered when planning to design and conduct a mixed methods study. Written for novice researchers, this is a very accessible discussion of how to apply the concepts from the field of mixed methods research to a mixed methods research study.

4. **Hesse-Biber, S. N., & Johnson, R. B. (Eds.) (2015).** *The Oxford handbook of multimethod and mixed methods research inquiry.* **Oxford, UK: Oxford University Press.**

- In this new handbook, Hesse-Biber and Johnson assembled authors from around the world and across disciplines to write about state-of-the-art perspectives on a wide range of standard and cutting-edge mixed methods research topics.

* The key resource is available at the following website: http://study.sagepub.com/planoclark.

REFERENCES

Alise, M. A., & Teddlie, C. (2010). A continuation of the paradigm wars? Prevalence rates of methodological approaches across the social/behavioral sciences. *Journal of Mixed Methods Research, 4*(2), 103–126.

Andrew, S., & Halcomb, E. J. (Eds.). (2009). *Mixed methods research for nursing and the health sciences*. Chichester, West Sussex, UK: Wiley-Blackwell.

Ayres, L. (2008). Grand theory. In L. M. Given (Ed.), *The SAGE encyclopedia of qualitative research methods* (pp. 374–375). Thousand Oaks, CA: Sage.

Bamberger, M., Rao, V., & Woolcock, M. (2010). Using mixed methods in monitoring and evaluation. In A. Tashakkori & C. Teddlie (Eds.), *SAGE handbook of mixed methods in social & behavioral research* (2nd ed., pp. 613–641). Thousand Oaks, CA: Sage.

Baran, M. (2010). Teaching multi-methodology research courses to doctoral students. *International Journal of Multiple Research Approaches, 4*(1), 19–27.

Bazeley, P. (2009). Integrating data analysis in mixed methods research. *Journal of Mixed Methods Research, 3*(3), 203–207.

Bazeley, P. (2010). Book review [Review of the book *The mixed methods reader,* by V. L. Plano Clark & J. W. Creswell (Eds.)]. *Journal of Mixed Methods Research, 4*(1), 79–81.

Bazeley, P., & Kemp, L. (2012). Mosaics, triangles, and DNA: Metaphors for integrated analysis in mixed methods research. *Journal of Mixed Methods Research, 6*(1), 55–72.

Becher, T., & Trowler, P. R. (2001). *Academic tribes and territories* (2nd ed.). Buckingham, UK: The Society for Research into Higher Education and Open University Press.

Bergman, M. M. (Ed.). (2008). *Advances in mixed methods research*. London: Sage.

Biddle, C., & Schafft, K. A. (2014). Axiology and anomaly in the practice of mixed methods work: Pragmatism, valuation, and the transformative paradigm. *Journal of Mixed Methods Research*. Advance online publication. doi:10.1177/1558689814533157

Biesta, G. (2010). Pragmatism and the philosophical and theoretical foundations of mixed methods research. In A. Tashakkori & C. Teddlie (Eds.), *SAGE handbook of mixed methods in social & behavioral research* (2nd ed., pp. 95–117). Thousand Oaks, CA: Sage.

Blakely, G., Skirton, H., Cooper, S., Allum, P., & Nelmes, P. (2010). Use of educational games in the health professions: A mixed-methods study of educators' perspectives in the UK. *Nursing and Health Sciences, 12,* 27–32.

Bradt, J., Burns, D. S., & Creswell, J. W. (2013). Mixed methods research in music therapy research. *Journal of Music Therapy, 50*(2), 123–148.

Brady, B., & O'Regan, C. (2009). Meeting the challenge of doing an RCT evaluation of youth mentoring in Ireland: A journey in mixed methods. *Journal of Mixed Methods Research, 3*(3), 265–280.

Brannen, J. (2005). Mixing methods: The entry of qualitative and quantitative approaches into the research process. *International Journal of Social Research Methodology, 8*(3), 173–184. doi:10.1080/13645570500154642

Brewer, J. (2003). Theory. In R. L. Miller & J. D. Brewer (Eds.), *The A-Z of social research* (pp. 324–327). London: Sage.

Brewer, J. D., & Hunter, A. (1989). *Multimethod research: A synthesis of styles.* Newbury Park, CA: Sage.

Bronfenbrenner, U. (1979). *The ecology of human development.* Cambridge, MA: Harvard University Press.

Brown, J. (2014). *Mixed methods research for TESOL.* Edinburgh, UK: Edinburgh University Press.

Bryman, A. (2006a). Integrating quantitative and qualitative research: How is it done? *Qualitative Research, 6*(1), 97–113.

Bryman, A. (2006b). Paradigm peace and the implications for quality. *International Journal of Social Research Methodology, 9*(2), 111–126.

Bryman, A. (2007). Barriers to integrating quantitative and qualitative research. *Journal of Mixed Methods Research, 1*(1), 8–22.

Bryman, A., Becker, S., & Semptik, J. (2008). Quality criteria for quantitative, qualitative and mixed methods research: A view from social policy. *International Journal of Social Research Methodology, 11*(4), 261–276.

Buck, G., Cook, K., Quigley, C., Eastwood, J., & Lucas, Y. (2009). Profiles of urban, low SES, African American girls' attitudes toward science: A sequential explanatory mixed methods study. *Journal of Mixed Methods Research, 3*(4), 386–410.

Burch, P., & Heinrich, C. J. (2015). *Mixed methods for policy research and program evaluation.* Thousand Oaks, CA: Sage.

Bush, E., Hux, K., Zickefoose, S., Simanek, G., Holmberg, M., & Henderson, A. (2011). Learning and study strategies of students with traumatic brain injury: A mixed methods study. *Journal of Postsecondary Education and Disability, 24*(3), 231–250.

Camerino, O., Castañer, M., & Anguera, M. T. (Eds.). (2012). *Mixed methods research in the movement sciences: Case studies in sport, physical education and dance.* Abingdon, Oxon, UK: Routledge.

Cameron, R. (2010). Mixed methods in VET research: Usage and quality. *International Journal of Training Research, 8*(1), 25–39.

Cameron, R. (2011). Mixed methods research: The five Ps framework. *The Electronic Journal of Research Methods, 9*(2), 87–197.

Campbell, R., Patterson, D., & Bybee, D. (2011). Using mixed methods to evaluate a community intervention for sexual assault survivors: A methodological tale. *Violence Against Women, 17*(3), 376–388.

Caracelli, V. J., & Greene, J. C. (1997). Crafting mixed-method evaluation designs. In J. C. Greene & V. J. Caracelli (Eds.), Advances in mixed-method evaluation: The challenges and benefits of integrating diverse paradigms. *New Directions for Evaluation* (Vol. 74, pp. 19–32). San Francisco: Jossey-Bass.

Chankseliani, M. (2013). Rural disadvantage in Georgian higher education admissions: A mixed-methods study. *Comparative Education Review, 57*(3), 424–456.

Chen, H. T. (2006). A theory-driven evaluation perspective on mixed methods research. *Research in the Schools, 13*(1), 75–83.

Chilisa, B., & Tsheko, G. N. (2014). Mixed methods in indigenous research: Building relationships for sustainable intervention outcomes. *Journal of Mixed Methods Research, 8*(3), 222–233.

Christ, T. W. (2009). Designing, teaching, and evaluating two complementary mixed methods research courses. *Journal of Mixed Methods Research, 3*(4), 292–325.

Christ, T. W. (2010). Teaching mixed methods and action research: Pedagogical, practical, and evaluative considerations. In A. Tashakkori & C. Teddlie (Eds.), *SAGE handbook of mixed methods in social & behavioral research* (2nd ed., pp. 643–676). Thousand Oaks, CA: Sage.

Christ, T. W. (2013). The worldview matrix as a strategy when designing mixed methods research. *International Journal of Multiple Research Approaches, 7*(1), 110–118.

Christ, T. W. (2014). Scientific-based research and randomized controlled trials, the "gold" standard? Alternative paradigms and mixed methodologies. *Qualitative Inquiry, 20*(1), 72–80.

Collins, K. M. T., & O'Cathain, A. (2009). Ten points about mixed methods research to be considered by the novice researcher. *International Journal of Multiple Research Approaches, 3,* 2–7.

Collins, K. M. T., Onwuegbuzie, A. J., & Jiao, Q. G. (Eds.). (2010). *Toward a broader understanding of stress and coping: Mixed methods approaches.* Charlotte, NC: Information Age Publishing.

Collins, K. M. T., Onwuegbuzie, A. J., & Sutton, I. L. (2006). A model incorporating the rationale and purpose for conducting mixed methods research in special education and beyond. *Learning Disabilities: A Contemporary Journal, 4,* 67–100.

Cooper, C., O'Cathain, A., Hind, D., Adamson, J., Lawton, J., & Baird, W. (2014). Conducting qualitative research within Clinical Trials Units: Avoiding potential pitfalls. *Contemporary Clinical Trials, 38*(2), 338–343. doi:10.1016/j.cct.2014.06.002

Craig, S. L. (2011). Precarious partnerships: Designing a community needs assessment to develop a system of care for gay, lesbian, bisexual, transgender and questioning (GLBTQ) youths. *Journal of Community Practice, 19,* 274–291.

Creswell, J. W. (2009). Mapping the field of mixed methods research [Editorial]. *Journal of Mixed Methods Research, 3*(2), 95–108.

Creswell, J. W. (2010). Mapping the developing landscape of mixed methods research. In A. Tashakkori & C. Teddlie (Eds.), *SAGE handbook of mixed methods in social & behavioral research* (2nd ed., pp. 45–68). Thousand Oaks, CA: Sage.

Creswell, J. W. (2013). *Qualitative inquiry and research design: Choosing among five approaches* (3rd ed.). Thousand Oaks, CA: Sage.

Creswell, J. W. (2014). *Research design: Qualitative, quantitative, and mixed methods approaches* (4th ed.). Thousand Oaks, CA: Sage.

Creswell, J. W. (2015). *A concise introduction to mixed methods research.* Thousand Oaks, CA: Sage.

Creswell, J. W., Fetters, M. D., & Ivankova, N. V. (2004). Designing a mixed methods study in primary care. *Annals of Family Medicine, 2*(1), 7–12.

Creswell, J. W., Fetters, M. D., Plano Clark, V. L., & Morales, A. (2009). Mixed methods intervention trials. In S. Andrew & E. J. Halcomb (Eds.), *Mixed methods research for nursing and the health sciences* (pp. 161–180). Hoboken, NJ: Wiley-Blackwell.

Creswell, J. W., Goodchild, L. F., & Turner, P. (1996). Integrated qualitative and quantitative research: Epistemology, history, and designs. In J. C. Smart (Ed.), *Higher education: Handbook of theory and research* (Vol. 11, pp. 90–136). New York, NY: Agathon Press.

Creswell, J. W., Klassen, A. C., Plano Clark, V. L., & Smith, K. C. for the Office of Behavioral and Social Sciences Research. (2011, August). *Best practices for mixed methods research in the health sciences.* Washington, DC: National Institutes of Health. Retrieved from http://obssr.od.nih.gov/mixed_methods_research

Creswell, J. W., & Plano Clark, V. L. (2007). *Designing and conducting mixed methods research.* Thousand Oaks, CA: Sage.

Creswell, J. W., & Plano Clark, V. L. (2011). *Designing and conducting mixed methods research* (2nd ed.). Thousand Oaks, CA: Sage.

Creswell, J. W., Plano Clark, V. L., Gutmann, M., & Hanson, W. (2003). Advanced mixed methods research designs. In A. Tashakkori & C. Teddlie (Eds.), *Handbook of mixed methods in social & behavioral research* (pp. 209–240). Thousand Oaks, CA: Sage.

Creswell, J. W., & Tashakkori, A. (2007). Developing publishable mixed methods manuscripts [Editorial]. *Journal of Mixed Methods Research, 1*(2), 107–111.

Creswell, J. W., Tashakkori, A., Jensen, K. D., & Shapley, K. L. (2003). Teaching mixed methods research: Practices, dilemmas, and challenges. In A. Tashakkori & C. Teddlie (Eds.), *Handbook of mixed methods in social & behavioral research* (pp. 619–637). Thousand Oaks, CA: Sage.

Crotty, M. (1998). *The foundations of social research: Meaning and perspective in the research process.* Thousand Oaks, CA: Sage.

Curry, L., & Nunez-Smith, M. (2015). *Mixed methods in health sciences research: A practical primer.* Thousand Oaks, CA: Sage.

Curry, L. A., Nembhard, I. M., & Bradley, E. H. (2009). Qualitative and mixed methods provide unique contributions to outcomes research. *Circulation, 119,* 1442–1452.

Curry, L. A., O'Cathain, A., Plano Clark, V. L., Aroni, R., Fetters, M., & Berg, D. (2012). The role of group dynamics in mixed methods health sciences research teams. *Journal of Mixed Methods Research, 6*(1) 5–20.

Dahlberg, B., Wittink, M., & Gallo, J. (2010). Funding and publishing integrated studies: Writing effective mixed methods manuscripts and grant proposals. In A. Tashakkori & C. Teddlie (Eds.), *SAGE handbook of mixed methods in social & behavioral research* (2nd ed., pp. 775–802). Thousand Oaks, CA: Sage.

Dellinger, A. B., & Leech, N. L. (2007). Toward a unified validation framework in mixed methods research. *Journal of Mixed Methods Research, 1*(4), 309–332.

Denscombe, M. (2008). Communities of practice: A research paradigm for the mixed methods approach. *Journal of Mixed Methods Research, 2*(3), 270–283.

Denzin, N. K. (1978). *The research act: A theoretical introduction to sociological methods*. New York, NY: McGraw-Hill.

Drabble, S. J., O'Cathain, A., Thomas, K. J., Rudolph, A., & Hewison, J. (2014). Describing qualitative research undertaken with randomised controlled trials in grant proposals: A documentary analysis. *BMC Medical Research Methodology, 14*(1), 24–35. doi:10.1186/1471-2288-14-24

Dumbili, E. W. (2014). Use of mixed methods designs in substance research: A methodological necessity in Nigeria. *Quality and Quantity, 48*(5), 2841–2857.

Dupin, C. M., Debout, C., & Rothan-Tondeur, M. (2014). Mixed-method nursing research: "A public and its problems?" A commentary on French nursing research. *Policy, Politics, and Nursing Practice, 15*(1–2), 15–20.

Edwards, G. (2010). *Mixed-method approaches to social network analysis* [Discussion paper]. Southampton, UK: National Centre for Research Methods. Retrieved from http://eprints.ncrm.ac.uk/842

Eisinger, A., & Senturia, K. (2001). Doing community-driven research: A description of Seattle Partners for Healthy Communities. *Journal of Urban Health, 78*, 519–534.

Ellis, L. A., Marsh, H. W., & Craven, R. G. (2009). Addressing the challenges faced by early adolescents: A mixed-method evaluation of the benefits of peer support. *American Journal of Community Psychology, 44*, 54–75.

Evans, B. C., Belyea, M. J., Coon, D. W., & Ume, E. (2012). Activities of daily living in Mexican American caregivers: The key to continuing informal care. *Journal of Family Nursing, 18*, 439–466.

Evans, B. C., Belyea, M. J., & Ume, E. (2011). Mexican American males providing personal care for their mothers. *Hispanic Journal of Behavioral Sciences, 33*, 234–260.

Evans, B. C., Coon, D. W., & Ume, E. (2011). Use of theoretical frameworks as a pragmatic guide for mixed methods studies: A methodological necessity? *Journal of Mixed Methods Research, 5*(4), 276–292.

Farmer, J., & Knapp, D. (2008). Interpretation programs at a historic preservation site: A mixed methods study of long-term impact. *Journal of Mixed Methods Research, 2*(4), 340–361.

Farquhar, M. C., Ewing, G., & Booth, S. (2011). Using mixed methods to develop and evaluate complex interventions in palliative care research. *Palliative Medicine, 25*(8), 748–757.

Feilzer, M. Y. (2010). Doing mixed methods research pragmatically: Implications for the rediscovery of pragmatism as a research paradigm. *Journal of Mixed Methods Research, 4*(1), 6–16. doi:10.1177/1558689809349691

Fielding, N. (2008). Analytic density, postmodernism, and applied multiple research method. In. M. M. Bergman (Ed.), *Advances in mixed methods research*. London: Sage.

Flick, U., Garms-Homolová, V., Herrmann, W. J., Kuck, J., & Röhnsch, G. (2012). "I can't prescribe something just because someone asks for it...": Using mixed methods in the framework of triangulation. *Journal of Mixed Methods Research, 6*(2), 97–110. doi:10.1177/1558689812437183

Freshwater, D. (2007). Reading mixed methods research. *Journal of Mixed Methods Research, 1*(2), 134–146. doi:10.1177/1558689806298578

Freshwater, D., & Cahill, J. (2012). Why write? [Editorial]. *Journal of Mixed Methods Research, 6*(3), 151–153.

Freshwater, D., & Cahill, J. (2013). Paradigms lost and paradigms regained [Editorial]. *Journal of Mixed Methods Research, 7*(1), 3–5.

Freshwater, D., & Fisher, P. (2014). (Con) fusing commerce and science: Mixed methods research and the production of contextualized knowledge [Editorial]. *Journal of Mixed Methods Research, 8*(2), 111–114.

Gay, L. R., Mills, G. E., & Airasian, P. (2012). *Educational research: Competencies for analysis and applications* (10th ed.). Boston: Pearson Education.

Giddings, L. S., & Grant, B. M. (2007). A Trojan horse for positivism? A critique of mixed methods research. *Advances in Nursing Science, 30*(1), 52–60.

Giddings, L. S., & Grant, B. M. (2009). From rigour to trustworthiness: Validating mixed methods. In S. Andrew & E. J. Halcomb (Eds.), *Mixed methods research for nursing and the health sciences* (pp. 119–134). Chichester, UK: Wiley-Blackwell.

Gomez, A. (2014). New developments in mixed methods with vulnerable groups. *Journal of Mixed Methods Research, 8*(3), 317–320.

Grafton, J., Lillis, A. M., & Mahama, H. (2011). Mixed methods research in accounting. *Qualitative Research in Accounting and Management, 8*(1), 5–21.

Grbich, C. (2007). Editorial. *International Journal of Multiple Research Approaches, 1*(1), 2. doi:10.5172/mra.455.1.1.2

Greene, J. C. (2007). *Mixed methods in social inquiry*. San Francisco, CA: Jossey-Bass.

Greene, J. C. (2008). Is mixed methods social inquiry a distinct methodology? *Journal of Mixed Methods Research, 2*(1), 7–22.

Greene, J. C. (2010). Forward: Beginning the conversation. *International Journal of Multiple Research Approaches, 4*(1), 2–5.

Greene, J. C. (2012). Engaging critical issues in social inquiry by mixing methods. *American Behavioral Scientist, 56*(6), 755–773. doi:10.1177/0002764211433794

Greene, J. C., & Caracelli, V. J. (Eds.). (1997a). Advances in mixed-method evaluation: The challenges and benefits of integrating diverse paradigms. *New Directions for Evaluation, 74*. San Francisco: Jossey-Bass.

Greene, J. C., & Caracelli, V. J. (1997b). Defining and describing the paradigm issue in mixed-method evaluation. In J. C. Greene & V. J. Caracelli (Eds.), Advances in mixed-method evaluation: The challenges and benefits of integrating diverse paradigms. *New Directions for Evaluation* (Vol. 74, pp. 5–17). San Francisco: Jossey-Bass.

Greene, J. C., & Caracelli, V. J. (2003). Making paradigmatic sense of mixed methods practice. In A. Tashakkori & C. Teddlie (Eds.), *Handbook of mixed methods in social & behavioral research* (pp. 91–110). Thousand Oaks, CA: Sage.

Greene, J. C., Caracelli, V. J., & Graham, W. F. (1989). Toward a conceptual framework for mixed-method evaluation designs. *Educational Evaluation and Policy Analysis, 11*(3), 255–274.

Greene, J. C., & Hall, J. N. (2010). Dialectics and pragmatism: Being of consequence. In A. Tashakkori & C. Teddlie (Eds.), *SAGE handbook of mixed methods in social & behavioral research* (2nd ed., pp. 119–143). Thousand Oaks, CA: Sage.

Greysen, S. R., Allen, R., Lucas, G. I., Wang, E. A., & Rosenthal, M. S. (2012). Understanding transitions in care from hospital to homeless shelter: A mixed-methods, community-based participatory approach. *Journal of General Internal Medicine, 27*(11), 1484–1491.

Guest, G. (2013). Describing mixed methods research: An alternative to typologies. *Journal of Mixed Methods Research, 7*(2), 141–151.

Hall, B., & Howard, K. (2008). A synergistic approach: Conducting mixed methods research with typological and systematic design considerations. *Journal of Mixed Methods Research, 2*(3), 248–269.

Hanson, W. E., Creswell, J. W., Plano Clark, V. L., Petska, K. P., & Creswell, J. D. (2005). Mixed methods research designs in counseling psychology. *Journal of Counseling Psychology, 52*(2), 224–235.

Harden, A., & Thomas, J. (2010). Mixed methods and systematic reviews: Examples and emerging issues. In A. Tashakkori & C. Teddlie (Eds.), *SAGE handbook of mixed methods in social & behavioral research* (2nd ed., pp. 749–774). Thousand Oaks, CA: Sage.

Harper, C. E. (2011). Identity, intersectionality, and mixed-methods approaches. *New Directions for Institutional Research, 2011*(151), 103–115. doi:10.1002/ir.401

Harrison, R. L., & Reilly, T. M. (2011). Mixed methods designs in marketing research. *Qualitative Market Research: An International Journal, 14*(1), 7–26.

Harrits, G. S. (2011). More than method? A discussion of paradigm differences within mixed methods research. *Journal of Mixed Methods Research, 5*(2), 150–166. doi:10.1177/1558689811402506

Hart, L. C., Smith, S. Z., Swars, S. L., & Smith, M. E. (2009). An examination of research methods in mathematics education (1995-2005). *Journal of Mixed Methods Research, 3*(1), 26–41.

Hemmings, A. (2005). Great ethical divides: Bridging the gap between institutional review board and the researchers. *Educational Researcher, 35*(4), 12–18.

Hemmings, A., Beckett, G., Kennerly, S., & Yap, T. (2013). Building a community of research practice: Intragroup team social dynamics in interdisciplinary mixed methods. *Journal of Mixed Methods Research, 7*(3), 261–273.

Hesse-Biber, S. N. (2010a). Feminist approaches to mixed methods research. In A. Tashakkori & C. Teddlie (Eds.), *SAGE handbook of mixed methods in social & behavioral research* (2nd ed., pp.169–192). Thousand Oaks, CA: Sage.

Hesse-Biber, S. N. (2010b). *Mixed methods research: Merging theory with practice.* New York, NY: Guilford Press.

Hesse-Biber, S. (2012). Feminist approaches to triangulation: Uncovering subjugated knowledge and fostering social change in mixed methods research. *Journal of Mixed Methods Research, 6*(2), 137–146.

Hesse-Biber, S., & Johnson, R. B. (2013). Coming at things differently: Future directions of possible engagement with mixed methods research [Editorial]. *Journal of Mixed Methods Research, 7*(2), 103–109.

Hesse-Biber, S. N., & Johnson, R. B. (Eds.). (2015). *The Oxford handbook of multimethod and mixed methods research inquiry.* Oxford, UK: Oxford University Press.

Hesse-Biber, S. N., & Leavy, P. (Eds.) (2008). *The handbook of emergent methods.* New York, NY: Guilford Press.

Hesse-Biber, S. N., & Leavy, P. (2011). *The practice of qualitative research* (2nd ed.). Thousand Oaks, CA: Sage.

Hewitt, J. (2007). Ethical components of researcher: Researched relationships in qualitative interviewing. *Qualitative Health Research, 17,* 1149–1159.

Heyvaert, M., Hannes, K., Maes, B., & Onghena, P. (2013). Critical appraisal of mixed methods studies. *Journal of Mixed Methods Research, 7*(4), 302–327. doi:10.1177/1558689813479449

Heyvaert, M., Maes, B., & Onghena, P. (2013). Mixed methods research synthesis: Definition, framework, and potential. *Quality & Quantity, 47,* 659–676.

Hinchey, P. H. (2008). *Action research: Primer.* New York, NY: Peter Lang.

Hodgkin, S. (2008). Telling it all: A story of women's social capital using a mixed methods approach. *Journal of Mixed Methods Research, 2*(3), 296–316.

Holtgraves, T. (1992). The linguistic realization of face management: Implications for language production and comprehension, person perception, and cross-cultural communication. *Social Psychology Quarterly, 55*(2), 141–159.

Howe, K. R. (2004). A critique of experimentalism. *Qualitative Inquiry, 10,* 42–61.

Howe, K. R. (2011). Mixed methods, mixed causes? *Qualitative Inquiry, 17*(2), 166–171. doi:10.1177/1077800410392524

Hurtado, S. (2012, April). *Reflections of a mixed methods researcher: Getting educated and educating others in defining quality in mixed methods.* Paper presented at the annual meeting of the American Educational Research Association, Vancouver, British Columbia, Canada.

Islam, F., & Oremus, M. (2014). Mixed methods immigrant mental health research in Canada: A systematic review. *Journal of Immigrant and Minority Health, 16*(6), 1284–1289.

Israel, B. A., Schulz, A. J., Parker, E. A., & Becker, A. B. (2001). Community-based participatory research: Policy recommendations for promoting a partnership approach in health research. *Education for Health: Change in Learning & Practice, 14*(2), 182–197.

Ivankova, N. V. (2010). Teaching and learning mixed methods research in computer-mediated environment: Educational gains and challenges. *International Journal of Multiple Research Approaches, 4*(1), 49–65.

Ivankova, N. V. (2014). Implementing quality criteria in designing and conducting a sequential QUAN→QUAL mixed methods study of student engagement with learning applied research methods online. *Journal of Mixed Methods Research, 8*(1), 25–51.

Ivankova, N. V. (2015). *Mixed methods applications in action research: From methods to community action.* Thousand Oaks, CA: Sage.

Ivankova, N. V., Creswell, J. W., & Stick, S. (2006). Using mixed methods sequential explanatory design: From theory to practice. *Field Methods, 18*(1), 3–20.

Ivankova, N. V., & Kawamura, Y. (2010). Emerging trends in the utilization of integrated designs in the social, behavioral, and health sciences. In A. Tashakkori & C. Teddlie (Eds.), *SAGE handbook of mixed methods in social and behavioral research* (2nd ed., pp. 581–611). Thousand Oaks, CA: Sage.

Ivankova, N. V., & Plano Clark, V. L. (2014, April). *Introducing a new mixed methods research I course: A practical guide to the field of mixed methods research.* Paper presented at the annual meeting of the American Educational Research Association, Philadelphia, PA.

Ivankova, N. V., & Plano Clark, V. L. (2015, April). *Developing a pedagogical approach for a new Mixed Methods Research I course as a guide to the complexity and nuances of the mixed methods research field.* Paper presented at the annual meeting of the American Educational Research Association, Chicago, IL.

Jang, E. E., McDougall, D. E., Pollon, D., Herbert, M., & Russell, P. (2008). Integrative mixed methods data analytic strategies in research on school success in challenging circumstances. *Journal of Mixed Methods Research, 2*(3), 221–247.

Jang, E. E., Wagner, M., & Park, G. (2014). Mixed methods research in language testing and assessment. *Annual Review of Applied Linguistics, 34,* 123–153.

Jick, T. D. (1979). Mixing qualitative and quantitative methods: Triangulation in action. *Administrative Science Quarterly, 24,* 602–611.

Johnson, R. B. (2012). Dialectical pluralism and mixed research. *American Behavioral Scientist, 56*(6), 751–754. doi:10.1177/0002764212442494

Johnson, R. B., McGowan, M. W., & Turner, L. A. (2010). Grounded theory in practice: Is it inherently a mixed method? *Research in the Schools, 17*(2), 65–78.

Johnson, R. B., & Onwuegbuzie, A. J. (2004). Mixed methods research: A research paradigm whose time has come. *Educational Researcher, 33*(7), 14–26.

Johnson, R. B., Onwuegbuzie, A. J., Tucker, S., & Icenogle, M. L. (2014). Conducting mixed methods research using dialectical pluralism and social psychological strategies. In P. Leavy (Ed.), *The Oxford handbook of qualitative research* (pp. 557–578), New York, NY: Oxford University Press.

Johnson, R. B., Onwuegbuzie, A. J., & Turner, L. A. (2007). Toward a definition of mixed methods research. *Journal of Mixed Methods Research, 1*(2), 112–133.

Johnson, R. B., & Turner, L. A. (2003). Data collection strategies in mixed methods research. In A. Tashakkori & C. Teddlie (Eds.), *Handbook of mixed methods in social & behavioral research* (pp. 297–319). Thousand Oaks, CA: Sage.

Jones-Harris, A. R. (2010). Are chiropractors in the UK primary healthcare or primary contact practitioners? A mixed methods study. *Chiropractic & Osteopathy, 18*(1), 28. doi:10.1186/1746-1340-18-28

Kawamura, Y., Ivankova, N., Kohler, C., & Perumean-Chaney, S. (2009). Utilizing mixed methods to assess parasocial interaction of one entertainment–education program audience. *International Journal of Multiple Research Approaches, 3*(1), 88–104.

Kim, K. H. (2014). Community-involved learning to expand possibilities for vulnerable children: A critical communicative, Sen's capability, and action research approach. *Journal of Mixed Methods Research, 8*(3), 308–316.

Kohrt, B. A. (2009). Vulnerable social groups in post-conflict settings: A mixed methods policy analysis. *Intervention, 7*(3), 239–264.

Koshy, E., Koshy, V., & Waterman, H. (2011). *Action research in healthcare.* Thousand Oaks, CA: Sage.

Krein, S. L., Kowalski, C. P., Damschroder, L., Forman, J., Kaufman, S. R., & Saint, S. (2008). Preventing ventilator-associated pneumonia in the United States: A multicenter mixed-methods study. *Infection Control and Hospital Epidemiology, 29*(10), 933–940.

Kroll, T., & Neri, M. T. (2005). Using mixed methods in disability and rehabilitation research. *Rehabilitation Nursing, 30*(3), 106–113.

Lanier, M. M., & Briggs, L. T. (2013). *Research methods in criminal justice and criminology: A mixed methods approach.* Oxford, UK: Oxford University Press.

Lee, Y. J., & Greene, J. (2007). The predictive validity of an ESL placement test: A mixed methods approach. *Journal of Mixed Methods Research, 1*(4), 366–389.

Leech, N. L. (2010). Interviews with the early developers of mixed methods research. In A. Tashakkori & C. Teddlie (Eds.), *SAGE handbook of mixed methods in social & behavioral research* (2nd ed., pp. 253–272). Thousand Oaks, CA: Sage.

Leech, N. L., Dellinger, A. B., Brannagan, K. B., & Tanaka, H. (2010). Evaluating mixed research studies: A mixed methods approach. *Journal of Mixed Methods Research, 4*(1), 17–31.

Leech, N. L., & Onwuegbuzie, A. J. (2009). A typology of mixed methods research designs. *Quality & Quantity, 43*(2), 265–275.

Leech, N. L., & Onwuegbuzie, A. J. (2010). The journey: From where we started to where we hope to go [Editorial]. *International Journal of Multiple Research Approaches, 4*(1), 73–88.

Lietz, C. A. (2009). Establishing evidence for strengths-based interventions? Reflections from social work's research conference [Editorial]. *Social Work, 54*(1), 85–87.

Lin, Y.-C., Liu, T.-C., & Chu, C.-C. (2011). Implementing clickers to assist learning in science lectures: The clicker-assisted conceptual change model. *Australasian Journal of Educational Technology, 27*(6), 979–996.

Lincoln, Y. S., & Guba, E. G. (1985). *Naturalistic inquiry.* Beverly Hills, CA: Sage.

Luck, L., Jackson, D., & Usher, K. (2006). Case study: A bridge across the paradigms. *Nursing Inquiry, 13*(2), 103–109.

Maramba, D. C., & Museus, S. D. (2011). The utility of using mixed-methods and intersectionality approaches in conducting research on Filipino American students' experiences with the campus climate and on sense of belonging. *New Directions for Institutional Research, 2011*(151), 93–101. doi:10.1002/ir.401

Marti, T. S., & Mertens, D. M. (2014). Mixed methods research with groups at risk: New developments and key debates [Editorial]. *Journal of Mixed Methods Research, 8*(3), 207–211.

Mason, J. (2006). Mixing methods in a qualitatively driven way. *Qualitative Research, 6*(1), 9–25.

Maxwell, J. A. (2011). Paradigms or toolkits? Philosophical and methodological positions as heuristics for mixed methods research. *Midwest Educational Research Journal, 24*(2), 27–30.

Maxwell, J. A. (2013). *Qualitative research design: An interactive approach* (3rd ed.). Thousand Oaks, CA: Sage.

Maxwell, J. A. (2015). Expanding the history and range of mixed methods research. *Journal of Mixed Methods Research.* Advance online publication. doi:10.1177/1558689815571132

Maxwell, J. A., & Loomis, D. M. (2003). Mixed methods design: An alternative approach. In A. Tashakkori & C. Teddlie (Eds.), *Handbook of mixed methods in social & behavioral research* (pp. 241–271). Thousand Oaks, CA: Sage.

Maxwell, J. A., & Mittapalli, K. (2008). Theory. In L. M. Given (Ed.), *The SAGE encyclopedia of qualitative research methods* (pp. 877–881). Thousand Oaks, CA: Sage.

Maxwell, J. A., & Mittapalli, K. (2010). Realism as a stance for mixed methods research. In A. Tashakkori & C. Teddlie (Eds.), *SAGE handbook of mixed methods in social & behavioral research* (2nd ed., pp. 145–167). Thousand Oaks, CA: Sage.

Mayoh, J., Bond, C. S., & Todres, L. (2012). An innovative mixed methods approach to studying the online health information seeking experiences of adults with chronic health conditions. *Journal of Mixed Methods Research, 6*(1), 21–33.

Mayoh, J., & Onwuegbuzie, A. J. (2015). Toward a conceptualization of mixed methods phenomenological research. *Journal of Mixed Methods Research, 9*(1), 91–107.

McClelland, S. I. (2014). "What do you mean when you say that you are sexually satisfied?" A mixed methods study. *Feminism & Psychology, 24*(1), 74–96.

McLeroy, K. R., Bibeau, D., Steckler, A., & Glanz, K. (1988). An ecological perspective on health promotion programs. *Health Education Quarterly, 15,* 351–377.

McNiff, J., & Whitehead, J. (2011). *All you need to know about action research* (2nd ed.). London: Sage.

Mertens, D. M. (2003). Mixed methods and the politics of human research: The transformative-emancipatory perspective. In A. Tashakkori & C. Teddlie (Eds.), *Handbook of mixed methods in social & behavioral research* (pp. 135–164). Thousand Oaks, CA: Sage.

Mertens, D. M. (2007). Transformative paradigm: Mixed methods and social justice. *Journal of Mixed Methods Research, 1*(3), 212–225.

Mertens, D. M. (2011). Publishing mixed methods research [Editorial]. *Journal of Mixed Methods Research, 5*(1), 3–6.

Mertens, D. M. (2013). Emerging advances in mixed methods: Addressing social justice [Editorial]. *Journal of Mixed Methods Research, 7*(3), 215–218.

Mertens, D. M. (2015). Mixed methods and wicked problems [Editorial]. *Journal of Mixed Methods Research, 9*(1), 3–6.

Mertens, D. M., Bledsoe, K. L., Sullivan, M., & Wilson, A. (2010). Utilization of mixed methods for transformative purposes. In A. Tashakkori & C. Teddlie (Eds.), *SAGE handbook of mixed methods in social & behavioral research* (2nd ed., pp. 193–214). Thousand Oaks, CA: Sage.

Mertens, D. M., & Hesse-Biber, S. (2012). Triangulation and mixed methods research: Provocative positions [Editorial]. *Journal of Mixed Methods Research, 6*(2), 75–79.

Miall, C. E., & March, K. (2005). Open adoption as a family form: Community assessments and social support. *Journal of Family Issues, 26*(3), 380–410.

Miller, W. L., & Crabtree, B. F. (2005). Clinical research. In N. Denzin & Y. Lincoln (Eds.), *The SAGE handbook of qualitative research* (3rd ed., pp. 605–639). Thousand Oaks, CA: Sage.

Mitchell, B. A. (2010). Happiness in midlife parental roles: A contextual mixed methods analysis. *Family Relations, 59,* 326–339.

Molina-Azorín, J. F. (2011). The use and added value of mixed methods in management research. *Journal of Mixed Methods Research, 5*(1), 7–24.

Morgan, D. L. (2007). Paradigms lost and pragmatism regained: Methodological implications of combining qualitative and quantitative methods. *Journal of Mixed Methods Research, 1*(1), 48–76.

Morgan, D. L. (2014). *Integrating qualitative and quantitative methods: A pragmatic approach*. Thousand Oaks, CA: Sage.

Morse, J. M. (1991). Approaches to qualitative-quantitative methodological triangulation. *Nursing Research, 40*(1), 120–123.

Morse, J. M. (2003). Principles of mixed methods and multimethod research design. In A. Tashakkori & C. Teddlie (Eds.), *Handbook of mixed methods in social & behavioral research* (pp. 189–208). Thousand Oaks, CA: Sage.

Morse, J. M. (2007). Ethics in action: Ethical principles for doing qualitative research. *Qualitative Health Research, 17*(8), 1003–1005.

Morse, J. M., & Niehaus, L. (2009). *Mixed method design: Principles and procedures*. Walnut Creek, CA: Left Coast Press.

Moubarac, J.-C., Cargo, M., Receveur, O., & Daniel, M. (2012). Describing the situational contexts of sweetened product consumption in a Middle Eastern Canadian community: Application of a mixed method design. *PLoS ONE 7*(9), e44738. doi:10.1371/journal.pone.0044738

Nastasi, B. K., & Hitchcock, J. (2016). *Mixed methods research and culture-specific interventions: Program design and evaluation*. Thousand Oaks, CA: Sage.

Nastasi, B. K., Hitchcock, J. H., & Brown, L. M. (2010). An inclusive framework for conceptualizing mixed methods design typologies: Moving toward fully integrated synergetic research models. In A. Tashakkori & C. Teddlie (Eds.), *SAGE handbook of mixed methods in social & behavioral research* (2nd ed., pp. 305–338). Thousand Oaks, CA: Sage.

Nastasi, B. K., Hitchcock, J. H., Sarkar, S., Burkholder, G., Varjas, K., & Jayasena, A. (2007). Mixed methods in intervention research: Theory to adaptation. *Journal of Mixed Methods Research, 1*(2), 164–182.

National Commission for the Protection of Human Subjects of Biomedical and Behavioral Research. (1979). *The Belmont Report: Ethical principles and guidelines for the protection of human subjects of research*. Washington, DC: U.S. Department of Health and Human Services: Retreived from http://www.hhs.gov/ohrp/human-subjects/guidance/belmont.html

Neuman, W. L. (2011). *Social research methods: Qualitative and quantitative approaches* (7th ed.). Boston, MA: Pearson Education.

Newman, I., & Ramlo, S. (2010). Using Q methodology and Q factor analysis in mixed methods research. In A. Tashakkori & C. Teddlie (Eds.), *SAGE handbook of mixed methods in social & behavioral research* (2nd ed., pp. 505–530). Thousand Oaks, CA: Sage.

Newman, I., Ridenour, C. S., Newman, C., & DeMarco, Jr., G. M. P. (2003). A typology of research purposes and its relationship to mixed methods. In A. Tashakkori & C. Teddlie (Eds.), *Handbook of mixed methods in social & behavioral research* (pp. 167–188). Thousand Oaks, CA: Sage.

Nilsen, A., & Brannen, J. (2010). The use of mixed methods in biographical research. In A. Tashakkori & C. Teddlie (Eds.), *SAGE handbook of mixed methods in social & behavioral research* (2nd ed., pp. 677–696). Thousand Oaks, CA: Sage.

Oakley, A. (1998). Gender, methodology and peoples ways of knowing: Some problems with feminism and the paradigm debate in social science. *Sociology, 32*(4), 707–731. doi:10.1177/0038038598032004005

O'Cathain, A. (2010). Assessing the quality of mixed methods research: Toward a comprehensive framework. In A. Tashakkori & C. Teddlie (Eds.), *SAGE handbook of mixed methods in social & behavioral research* (2nd ed., pp. 531–555). Thousand Oaks, CA: Sage.

O'Cathain, A., Murphy, E., & Nicholl, J. (2007). Why, and how, mixed methods research is undertaken in health services research in England: A mixed methods study. *BMC Health Services Research, 7*(85). doi:10.1186/1472-6963-7-85

O'Cathain, A., Murphy, E., & Nicholl, J. (2008). The quality of mixed methods studies in health services research. *Journal of Health Services Research Policy, 13*(2), 92–98.

Olson, B. D., & Jason, L. A. (2015). Participatory mixed methods research (PMMR). In S. N. Hesse-Biber & R. B. Johnson (Eds.), *The Oxford handbook of multimethod and mixed methods research inquiry* (pp. 393–405). Oxford, UK: Oxford University Press.

Onwuegbuzie, A. J., & Frels, R. K. (2013). Introduction: Toward a new research philosophy for addressing social justice issues: Critical dialectical pluralism 1.0. *International Journal of Multiple Research Approaches, 7*(1), 9–26.

Onwuegbuzie, A. J., Frels, R. K., Collins, K. M. T., & Leech, N. L. (2013). Conclusion: A four-phase model for teaching and learning mixed research. [Editorial]. *International Journal of Multiple Research Approaches, 7*(1), 133–156.

Onwuegbuzie, A. J., & Johnson, R. B. (2006). The validity issue in mixed research. *Research in the Schools, 13*(1), 48–63.

Onwuegbuzie, A. J., & Leech, N. L. (2006). Linking research questions to mixed methods data analysis procedures. *The Qualitative Report, 11*(3), 474–498.

Onwuegbuzie, A. J., Leech, N. L., Murtonen, M., & Tähtinen, J. (2010). Utilizing mixed methods in teaching environments to reduce statistics anxiety. *International Journal of Multiple Research Approaches, 4*(1), 28–39.

Onwuegbuzie, A. J., Rosli, R., Ingram, J. M., & Frels, R. K. (2014). A critical dialectical pluralistic examination of the lived experience of select women doctoral students. *The Qualitative Report, 19*(3), 1–35.

Padgett, D. (2012). *Qualitative and mixed methods in public health*. Thousand Oaks, CA: Sage.

Papadimitriou, A., Ivankova, N., & Hurtado, S. (2013). Addressing challenges of conducting quality mixed methods studies in higher education. In J. Huisman & M. Tight (Eds.), *Theory and method in higher education research: International perspectives on higher education research* (Vol. 9, pp. 133–153). London, UK: Emerald Group Publishing Limited.

Parmelee, J. H., Perkins, S. C., & Sayre, J. J. (2007). "What about people our age?" Applying qualitative and quantitative methods to uncover how political ads alienate college students. *Journal of Mixed Methods Research, 1*(2), 183–199.

Patton, M. Q. (2008). *Utilization-focused evaluation* (4th ed.). Thousand Oaks, CA: Sage.

Peterson, J. C., Czajkowski, S., Charlson, M. E., Link, A. R., Wells, M. T., Isen, A. M., . . . Jobe, J. B. (2013). Translating basic behavioral and social science research to clinical application: The EVOLVE mixed methods approach. *Journal of Consulting and Clinical Psychology, 81*(2), 217–230.

Phillips, J., & Davidson, P. M. (2009). Action research as a mixed methods design: A palliative approach in residential aged care. In S. Andrew & E. J. Halcomb (Eds.), *Mixed methods research for nursing and the health sciences* (pp. 195–216). Hoboken, NJ: Wiley-Blackwell.

Plano Clark, V. L. (2005). Cross-disciplinary analysis of the use of mixed methods in physics education research, counseling psychology, and primary care. Available from ProQuest Dissertations and Theses database. (UMI No. 3163998)

Plano Clark, V. L. (2010). The adoption and practice of mixed methods: U.S. trends in federally funded health-related research. *Qualitative Inquiry, 16*(6), 428–440.

Plano Clark, V. L., Anderson, N., Zhou, Y., Wertz, J., Schumacher, K., & Miaskowski, C. (2014). Conceptualizing longitudinal mixed methods designs:

A methodological review of health sciences research. *Journal of Mixed Methods Research*. Advance online publication. doi:10.1177/1558689814543563

Plano Clark, V. L., & Badiee, M. (2010). Research questions in mixed methods research. In A. Tashakkori & C. Teddlie (Eds.), *SAGE handbook of mixed methods in social & behavioral research* (2nd ed., pp. 275–304). Thousand Oaks, CA: Sage.

Plano Clark, V. L., & Creswell, J. W. (Eds.). (2008). *The mixed methods reader.* Thousand Oaks, CA: Sage.

Plano Clark, V. L., Huddleston-Casas, C. A., Churchill, S. L., Green, D. O., & Garrett, A. L. (2008). Mixed methods approaches in family science research. *Journal of Family Issues, 29*(11), 1543–1566.

Plano Clark, V. L., Schumacher, K., West, C., Edrington, J., Dunn, L. B., Harzstark, A., . . . Miaskowski, C. (2013). Practices for embedding an interpretive qualitative approach within a randomized clinical trial. *Journal of Mixed Methods Research, 7*(3), 219–242.

Plowright, D. (2011). *Using mixed methods: Frameworks for an integrated methodology.* London: Sage.

Poth, C. (2014). What constitutes effective learning experiences in a mixed methods research course? An examination from the student perspective. *International Journal of Multiple Research Approaches, 8*(1), 74–86.

Preissle, J., Glover-Kudon, R. M., Rohan, E. A., Boehm, J. E., & DeGroff, A. (2015). Putting ethics on the mixed methods map. In S. N. Hesse-Biber & R. B. Johnson (Eds.), *The Oxford handbook of multimethod and mixed methods research inquiry* (pp. 144–166). Oxford, UK: Oxford University Press.

Quan-Haase, A. (2007). University students' local and distant social ties: Using and integrating modes of communication on campus. *Information, Communication & Society, 10,* 671–693. doi:10.1080/13691180701658020

Rallis, S. F., & Rossman, G. B. (2003). Mixed methods in evaluation contexts: A pragmatic framework. In A. Tashakkori & C. Teddlie (Eds.), *Handbook of mixed methods in social & behavioral research* (pp. 491–512). Thousand Oaks, CA: Sage.

Reason, P., & Bradbury, H. (2008). Introduction. In P. Reason & H. Bradbury (Eds.), *The SAGE handbook of action research: Participative inquiry and practice* (2nd ed., pp. 1–10). Thousand Oaks, CA: Sage.

Reichardt, C. S., & Cook, T. D. (1979). Beyond qualitative versus quantitative methods. In T. D. Cook & C. S. Reichardt (Eds.), *Qualitative and quantitative methods in evaluation research* (pp. 7–32). Beverly Hills, CA: Sage.

Ridenour, C. S., & Newman, I. (2008). *Mixed methods research: Exploring the interactive continuum* (2nd ed.). Carbondale: Southern Illinois University Press.

Roberts, L. D., & Povee, K. (2014). A brief measure of attitudes toward mixed methods research in psychology. *Frontiers in Psychology, 5,* 1–10. doi:10.3389/fpsyg.2014.01312

Rosenfield, P. (1992). The potential of transdisciplinary research for sustaining and extending linkages between the health and social sciences. *Social Science and Medicine, 35*(11), 1343–1357.

Ross, A., & Onwuegbuzie, A. J. (2012). Prevalence of mixed methods research in mathematics education. *The Mathematics Educator, 22*(1), 84–113.

Rossi, P. H., Lipsey, M. W., & Freeman, H. E. (2004). *Evaluation: A systematic approach* (7th ed.). Thousand Oaks, CA: Sage.

Rudd, A., & Johnson, R. B. (2010). A call for more mixed methods in sport management research. *Sport Management Review, 13,* 14–24.

Ruffin, M. T., IV, Creswell, J. W., Jimbo, M., & Fetters, M. D. (2009). Factors influencing choices for colorectal cancer screening among previously unscreened African and Caucasian Americans: Findings from a triangulation mixed methods investigation. *Journal of Community Health, 34*(2), 79–89.

Saint Arnault, D., & Fetters, M. D. (2011). R01 funding for mixed methods research: Lessons learned from the "Mixed-Method Analysis of Japanese Depression" project. *Journal of Mixed Methods Research, 5*(4), 309–329.

Sale, J. E., Lohfeld, L. H., & Brazil, K. (2002). Revisiting the quantitative-qualitative debate: Implications for mixed-methods research. *Quality & Quantity, 36,* 43–53.

Sandelowski, M. (2000). Combining qualitative and quantitative sampling, data collection, and analysis techniques in mixed-methods studies. *Research in Nursing & Health, 23,* 246–255.

Sandelowski, M. (2012). The weakness of the strong/weak comparison of modes of inquiry [Editorial]. *Research in Nursing & Health, 35,* 325–327.

Sandelowski, M., Voils, C. I., Leeman, J., & Crandell, J. L. (2012). Mapping the mixed methods-mixed research synthesis terrain. *Journal of Mixed Methods Research, 6*(4), 317–331. doi:10.1177/1558689811427913

Schifferdecker, K. D., & Reed, V. A. (2009). Using mixed methods research in medical education: Basic guidelines for researchers. *Medical Education, 43,* 637–644.

Seltzer-Kelly, D., Westwood, S. J., & Peña-Guzman, D. M. (2012). A methodological self-study of quantitizing: Negotiating meaning and revealing multiplicity. *Journal of Mixed Methods Research, 6*(4), 258–274.

Shadish, W. R., Cook, T. D., & Campbell, D. T. (2002). *Experimental and quasi-experimental designs for generalized causal inference.* Boston, MA: Houghton Mifflin.

Shannon-Baker, P. (2015). Making paradigms meaningful in mixed methods research. *Journal of Mixed Methods Research.* Advance online publication. doi:10.1177/1558689815575861

Shepard, M. P., Orsi, A. J., Mahon, M. M., & Carroll, R. M. (2002). Mixed-methods research with vulnerable families. *Journal of Family Nursing, 8*(4), 334–352.

Shuayb, M. (2014). Appreciative inquiry as a method for participatory change in secondary schools in Lebanon. *Journal of Mixed Methods Research, 8*(3), 299–307.

Shulha, L. M., & Wilson, R. J. (2003). Collaborative mixed methods research. In A. Tashakkori & C. Teddlie (Eds.), *Handbook of mixed methods in social & behavioral research* (pp. 639–669). Thousand Oaks, CA: Sage.

Singh, E., Milne, S., & Hull, J. (2012). Use of mixed-methods case study to research sustainable tourism development in South Pacific SIDS. In K. F. Hyde, C. Ryan, & A. G. Woodside (Eds.), Field guide to case study research in tourism, hospitality and leisure. *Advances in Culture, Tourism and Hospitality Research* (Vol. 6, pp. 457–478). London, UK: Emerald Group Publishing Limited.

Small, M. L. (2011). How to conduct a mixed methods study: Recent trends in a rapidly growing literature. *Annual Review of Sociology, 37,* 57–86.

Smith, J. K. (1983). Quantitative versus qualitative research: An attempt to clarify the issue. *Educational Researcher, 12*(3), 6–13.

Song, M.-K., Sandelowski, M., & Happ, M. B. (2010). Current practices and emerging trends in conducting mixed methods intervention studies in the health sciences. In A. Tashakkori & C. Teddlie (Eds.), *SAGE handbook of mixed methods in social & behavioral research* (2nd ed., pp. 725–747). Thousand Oaks, CA: Sage.

Stake, R. E. (1995). *The art of case study research.* Thousand Oaks, CA: Sage.

Stange, K., Crabtree, B., & Miller, W. (2006). Publishing multimethod research. *Annals of Family Medicine, 4,* 292–294.

Stentz, J. E., Plano Clark, V. L., & Matkin, G. S. (2012). Applying mixed methods to leadership research: A review of current practices. *The Leadership Quarterly, 23,* 1173–1183.

Stokols, D. (1996). Translating social ecological theory into guidelines for community health promotion. *American Journal of Health Promotion, 10,* 282–298.

Sullivan, M., Derrett, S., Paul, C., Beaver, C., & Stace, H. (2014). Using mixed methods to build research capacity within the spinal cord injured population in New Zealand. *Journal of Mixed Methods Research, 8*(3), 234–244.

Swanson, S. C. (1992). A cross-disciplinary application of Greene, Caracelli and Graham's conceptual framework for mixed method evaluation (Doctoral dissertation). Available from ProQuest Dissertations and Theses database. (UMI No. 3344745)

Sweetman, D., Badiee, M., & Creswell, J. W. (2010). Use of the transformative framework in mixed methods studies. *Qualitative Inquiry, 16*(6), 441–454.

Tashakkori, A. (2009). Are we there yet? The state of the mixed methods community [Editorial]. *Journal of Mixed Methods Research, 3*(4), 287–291.

Tashakkori, A., & Creswell, J. W. (2007a). Exploring the nature of research questions in mixed methods research [Editorial]. *Journal of Mixed Methods Research, 1*(3), 207–211.

Tashakkori, A., & Creswell, J. W. (2007b). The new era of mixed methods [Editorial]. *Journal of Mixed Methods Research, 1*(1), 3–7.

Tashakkori, A., & Creswell, J. W. (2008). Mixed methodology across disciplines [Editorial]. *Journal of Mixed Methods Research, 2*(1), 3–6.

Tashakkori, A., & Teddlie, C. (1998). *Mixed methodology: Combining qualitative and quantitative approaches.* Thousand Oaks, CA: Sage.

Tashakkori, A., & Teddlie, C. (Eds.). (2003a). *Handbook of mixed methods in social & behavioral research.* Thousand Oaks, CA: Sage.

Tashakkori, A., & Teddlie, C. (2003b). The past and future of mixed methods research: From data triangulation to mixed model designs. In A. Tashakkori & C. Teddlie (Eds.), *Handbook of mixed methods in social & behavioral research* (pp. 671–701). Thousand Oaks, CA: Sage.

Tashakkori, A., & Teddlie, C. (2010a). Epilogue: Current developments and emerging trends in integrated research methodology. In A. Tashakkori & C. Teddlie (Eds.), *SAGE handbook of mixed methods in social & behavioral research* (2nd ed., pp. 803–826). Thousand Oaks, CA: Sage.

Tashakkori, A., & Teddlie, C. (Eds.). (2010b). *SAGE handbook of mixed methods in social & behavioral research* (2nd ed.). Thousand Oaks, CA: Sage.

Teddlie, C., & Tashakkori, A. (2003). Major issues and controversies in the use of mixed methods in the social and behavioral sciences. In A. Tashakkori & C. Teddlie (Eds.), *Handbook of mixed methods in social & behavioral research* (pp. 3–50). Thousand Oaks, CA: Sage.

Teddlie, C., & Tashakkori, A. (2006). A general typology of research designs featuring mixed methods. *Research in the Schools, 13*(1), 12–28.

Teddlie, C., & Tashakkori, A. (2009). *Foundations of mixed methods research: Integrating quantitative and qualitative approaches in the social and behavioral sciences*. Thousand Oaks, CA: Sage.

Teddlie, C., & Tashakkori, A. (2010). Overview of contemporary issues in mixed methods research. In A. Tashakkori & C. Teddlie (Eds.), *SAGE handbook of mixed methods in social & behavioral research* (pp. 1–41). Thousand Oaks, CA: Sage.

Thorndike, R. M., & Thorndike-Christ, T. M. (2011). *Measurement and evaluation in psychology and education* (8th ed.). Upper Saddle River, NJ: Pearson Education.

Van Ness, P. H., Fried, T. R., & Gill, T. M. (2011). Mixed methods for the interpretation of longitudinal gerontologic data: Insights from philosophical hermeneutics. *Journal of Mixed Methods Research, 5*(4), 293–308.

Wagner, K. D., Davidson, P. J., Pollini, R. A., Strathdee, S. A., Washburn, R., & Palinkas, L. A. (2012). Reconciling incongruous qualitative and quantitative findings in mixed methods research: Exemplars from research with drug using populations. *International Journal on Drug Policy, 23*(1), 54–61.

Weisner, T. S., (Ed.). (2005). *Discovering successful pathways in children's development: Mixed methods in the study of childhood and family life*. Chicago, IL: University of Chicago Press.

Wilson, A. T., & Winiarczyk, R. E. (2014). Mixed methods research strategies with deaf people: Linguistic and cultural challenges addressed. *Journal of Mixed Methods Research, 8*(3), 266–277.

Windsor, L. C. (2013). Using concept mapping in community-based participatory research: A mixed methods approach. *Journal of Mixed Methods Research, 7*(3), 274–293.

Yin, R. K. (2006). Mixed methods research: Are the methods genuinely integrated or merely parallel? *Research in the Schools, 13*(1), 41–47.

Yin, R. K. (2014). *Case study research: Design and methods* (5th ed.). Thousand Oaks, CA: Sage.

Zachariadis, M., Scott, S., & Barrett, M. (2013). Methodological implications of critical realism for mixed-methods research. *Management Information Systems, 37*(3), 855–879.

Zea, M. C., Aguilar-Pardo, M., Betancourt, F., Reisen, C., & Gonzales, F. (2014). Mixed methods with internally displaced Colombian gay and bisexual men and transwomen. *Journal of Mixed Methods Research, 8*(3), 212–221.

Zhou, Y., & Creswell, J. W. (2012). The use of mixed methods by Chinese scholars in East China: A case study. *International Journal of Multiple Research Approaches, 6*(1), 73–87.

INDEX

Brazil, K., 97
Bronfenbrenner, U., 14
Bryman, A., 90–91 (table), 97, 102–103
Buck, G., 6–7, 29, 37, 38, 40
  priority given to data by, 41
  sequential studies used by, 41
Burkholder, G., 158
Burns, D. S., 258 (table)
Bush, E., 147
Bybee, D., 278, 295–296

Cahill, J., 206, 208, 234
Cameron, R., 228, 240, 262 (table)
Campbell, R., 278, 295–296
Caracelli, V. J., 64 (table), 88 (table),
  102, 140, 200 (table)
  on theoretical framework, 144
Cargo, M., 124
Carroll, R. M., 227 (table)
Case studies, mixed methods,
  146–147
"Case study: A bridge across the
  paradigms," 158
Chankesliani, M., 227 (table)
Charlson, M. E., 69, 148
Chen, H. T., 204
Christ, T. W., 197, 254–255
Chu, C.-C., 146
Churchill, S. L., 261 (table)
Collins, K. M. T., 89 (table), 269, 279,
  280 (table), 296
Colorectal cancer screening choices
  study, 5, 7–9, 19–21
"Coming at things differently: Future
  directions of possible engagement
  with mixed methods research," 29
Communities of research practice, 57,
  62–63, 225, 264
Community-based participatory research
  (CBPR), 149, 224
Complementarity rationale, 81, 85, 87,
  88 (table)
Completeness rationale, 90 (table)
Complex Mixed and Multiple Method
  Designs, 113 (table)
Component mixed methods designs, 112
  (table)

Comprehensive framework for assessing
  quality of mixed methods research,
  173 (table)
Conceptual frameworks, 204
Conceptualization of mixed methods
  research, 9–10, 13
  See also Socio-ecological framework
  for field of mixed methods
  research
*Concise Introduction to Mixed Methods
  Research, A,* 215
Concurrent quan + qual design, 107,
  119–121
Concurrent timing, 39–40
Confirm and discover rationale, 91
  (table)
Constructivism, 196, 198–199 (table)
Construct validation, 168, 181
Content, mixed methods research, 5,
  16–17 (table), 16 (table), 18, 21,
  23–24
  future of, 293
Context rationale, 91 (table)
Contexts, disciplinary, 248, 253–254
Contexts, institutional, 249, 252–253
Contexts, interpersonal
  applied in mixed methods research
  practice, 240–243
  defined, 218, 219–220
  editorial and review board guidelines
  and, 219, 228–229
  examples, 229–234
  issues and debates about, 234–240
  major perspectives about, 221–229
  research ethics and, 219, 221–223
  research participant considerations
  and, 219, 223–225
  research team dynamics and, 219,
  225–228
  role in field of mixed methods
  research, 219–221
Contexts, mixed methods research, 5, 17
  (table), 19, 21, 24
  future of, 293–294
Contexts, personal, 193
  applied in mixed methods research
  practice, 210–213

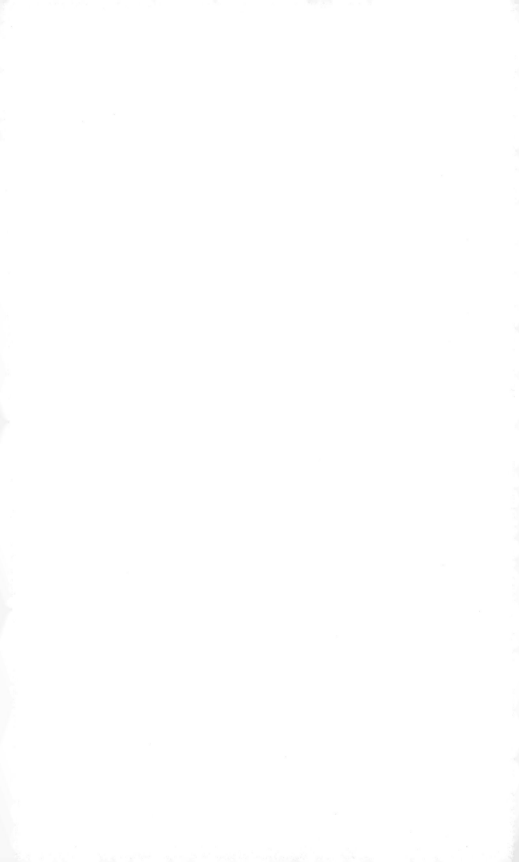